VETERINARY HEMATOLOGY
ATLAS OF COMMON DOMESTIC AND NON-DOMESTIC SPECIES

SECOND EDITION

VETERINARY HEMATOLOGY

ATLAS OF COMMON DOMESTIC AND NON-DOMESTIC SPECIES

SECOND EDITION

William J. Reagan

Armando R. Irizarry Rovira

Dennis B. DeNicola

WILEY-BLACKWELL

A John Wiley & Sons, Inc., Publication

First edition first published 1998
© 1998 Iowa State University Press
Second edition first published 2008
© 2008 Wiley-Blackwell

Blackwell Publishing was acquired by John Wiley & Sons in February 2007.
Blackwell's publishing program has been merged with Wiley's global Scientific,
Technical, and Medical business to form Wiley-Blackwell.

Editorial Office
2121 State Avenue, Ames, Iowa 50014-8300, USA

For details of our global editorial offices, for customer services, and for
information about how to apply for permission to reuse the copyright material in
this book, please see our website at www.wiley.com/wiley-blackwell.

Library of Congress Cataloging-in-Publication Data

Reagan, William J.
    Veterinary hematology: atlas of common domestic and non-domestic species /
William J. Reagan, Armando R. Irizarry Rovira, Dennis B. DeNicola. – 2nd ed.
        p. ; cm.
    Includes bibliographical references and index.
    ISBN 978-0-8138-2809-1 (alk. paper)
    1. Veterinary hematology–Atlases.   I. Irizarry Rovira, Armando R.
II. DeNicola, D. B.   III. Title.
    [DNLM: 1. Hematologic Diseases–veterinary–Atlases.   2. Animals, Domestic–
Atlases. SF 769.5 R287v 2008]
    SF769.5.R43 2008
    636.089'615–dc22
    2008011368

A catalogue record for this book is available from the U.S. Library of Congress.

Set in Times New Roman by SNP Best-set Typesetter Ltd., Hong Kong
Printed in Singapore by Markono Print Media Pte Ltd

5   2012

CONTENTS

Preface

The purpose of this book is to provide the fundamentals for recognizing the normal and abnormal morphological features of blood cells of the common domestic and non-domestic species. The first edition was limited to the morphology of the common domestic species, including dogs, cats, horses, ruminants, and llamas. This second edition has been greatly expanded to include the commonly used laboratory animal species, including rats (Sprague-Dawley), mice (CD1), nonhuman primates (cynomolgus monkey; *Macaca fascicularis*), ferrets, rabbits (New Zealand White), and guinea pigs. In addition, chapters on avian and reptilian hematology are also included. These chapters demonstrate the normal and abnormal morphology in many of the common pet avian and reptilian species. To accomplish this hematology review of the common domestic and non-domestic species, photomicrographs that show many of the common, as well as some of the less frequent, blood morphologic abnormalities are presented. A high number of the photomicrographs are of canine blood smears, but many of the abnormalities shown occur in other species as well. Those that are unique to one species are mentioned. Attempts were made to be as complete as possible, but clearly, not all abnormalities that can be found in the blood are shown. There is also a list of selected references provided that may be helpful in evaluating a morphological feature that is not described in this book. Throughout the book, in addition to the morphological features of the blood cells, some of the more common diseases or pathophysiological states in which these abnormalities may occur are mentioned. These lists of disease states are not always totally inclusive of all possible states in which these abnormalities may occur, and the readers are again referred to more complete treatises of hematology in the references.

Wright or Wright-Giemsa stains were used on the majority of blood smears that were photographed. If another stain was used, it is stated in the figure legend. If no stain is mentioned in the figure legend, the stain used was Wright or Wright-Giemsa. Other stains including Diff-Quik and other similar rapid stains are identified specifically as Diff-Quik stain or simply as "quick stain." The color reproductions of the cells were kept as consistent and as accurate as possible. The descriptions in the text and figure legends highlight these characteristics. However, depending on the exact type of stain used by the reader, the color of the blood cells may be slightly different from those described in the text. Some of the major differences in staining are described in Chapter 10.

The microscope objective that was used to take the photomicrographs is also listed in the figure legend. The objective is listed instead of the total original magnification in an attempt to make it easier to understand how a cell, inclusion, and so on would appear on the reader's microscope. The final magnification of most of the figures is similar, so that the figures with the same objective listed can be compared directly. Insets have been added to several figures, which may give a greater magnification of the cell or object of interest; these are marked appropriately.

This textbook should be useful to the novice and experienced hematologist alike. The glossary, which defines many of the terms used in the text, may be more useful to the novice. Two appendixes, which present methods used in the Purdue University Veterinary Teaching Hospital Clinical Pathology Laboratory for semiquantitation of some of the morphological abnormalities, may be useful to the novice as well as the experienced hematologist. These appendixes should be helpful guidelines for reproducibly recording morphological abnormalities that may be present in a blood smear.

Finally, we have many people to thank for their assistance in developing the second edition of the atlas. First and most important are our families, who provided us with the time and support to pursue this project. Special thanks go to our wives, Julie Clements-Reagan, Heather Irizarry, and Jan DeNicola. We also thank Julie Clements-Reagan again for her contribution to the graphic design of first edition, which is also retained in this edition. We thank Teresa Sanders and the technicians and clinical pathology residents of the Purdue University Veterinary Teaching Hospital Clinical Pathology Laboratory for suggestions on content, as well as help in acquiring the case material used in the first edition and again used in the second edition. We are thankful for the many avian and reptilian samples that non-domestic animal practitioners, such as Dr. Angela Lennox (Avian and Exotic Animal Clinic of Indianapolis, Indiana) and Dr. Alexander Wolf (Avian and Exotic Animal Clinic of Lafayette, Indiana), contributed over the past many years. Some additional material was obtained from glass slides that were submitted to the American Society for Veterinary Clinical Pathology annual slide review; those slides are identified as such in the legends. We thank the society and contributors for this material. Finally, we appreciate the support and opportunity that Wiley-Blackwell has given us to develop this resource.

ABOUT THE AUTHORS

WILLIAM J. REAGAN received his DVM degree from the College of Veterinary Medicine, Ohio State University, Columbus, and his PhD degree from the College of Veterinary Medicine and Biomedical Sciences, Colorado State University, Fort Collins. He is a Diplomate of the American College of Veterinary Pathologists. Dr. Reagan was formerly an associate professor of veterinary clinical pathology, Purdue University School of Veterinary Medicine, West Lafayette, Indiana, and is currently an associate research fellow at Pfizer, Inc., Groton, Connecticut.

ARMANDO R. IRIZARRY ROVIRA received his DVM and PhD degrees from the School of Veterinary Medicine, Purdue University. He is a Diplomate of the American College of Veterinary Pathologists and is currently a research advisor-pathologist at Eli Lilly and Company, Greenfield, Indiana, as well as an adjunct associate professor of veterinary anatomic and clinical pathology at Purdue University School of Veterinary Medicine, West Lafayette, Indiana.

DENNIS B. DENICOLA received his DVM degree from the School of Veterinary Medicine, Purdue University, and his PhD from Purdue University. He is a Diplomate of the American College of Veterinary Pathologists and was formerly a professor of veterinary clinical pathology, Purdue University. Dr. DeNicola currently is the chief veterinary educator at IDEXX Laboratories, Inc., Westbrook, Maine, and adjunct professor of veterinary clinical pathology at Purdue University.

VETERINARY HEMATOLOGY
ATLAS OF COMMON DOMESTIC AND NON-DOMESTIC SPECIES

SECOND EDITION

CHAPTER ONE

HEMATOPOIESIS

GENERAL FEATURES

All blood cells have a finite life span, but in normal animals, the number of cells in circulation is maintained at a fairly constant level. To accomplish this, cells in circulation need to be constantly replenished, which occurs via the production and release of cells from the bone marrow. Production sites in the bone marrow are commonly referred to as medullary sites.

In times of increased demand, production can also occur outside the bone marrow in sites such as spleen, liver, and lymph nodes. These sites are called extramedullary sites. In rodents, in the normal steady state, extramedullary production of blood cells occurs in the spleen.

Hematopoiesis, the production of blood cells, is a complex and highly regulated process. Some differences in hematopoiesis exist between species and are

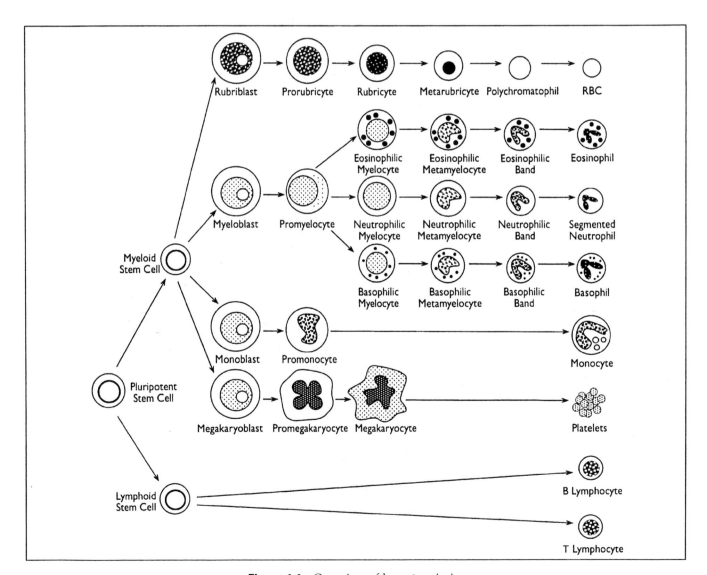

Figure 1.1 Overview of hematopoiesis.

beyond the scope of this text; readers are referred to the detailed coverage in some of the Selected References. The dog will be used to demonstrate some of the basic principles of hematopoiesis. All blood cells in the bone marrow arise from a common stem cell. This pluripotent stem cell gives rise to several stages of committed progenitor cells, which then differentiate into cells of the erythrocytic, granulocytic, megakaryocytic, and agranulocytic (monocytic and lymphocytic) lineages. The end result of this development process is the release of red blood cells, white blood cells, and platelets into the circulation. At the light microscopic level, without the use of immunocytochemistry or enzyme cytochemistry, it is impossible to accurately identify the early stem cells in the bone marrow, but the more differentiated stages of development can be identified and are graphically depicted in Figure 1.1.

Figure 1.2 shows a histological section of a bone marrow core biopsy from an adult dog. Note that there is a mixture of approximately 50 percent hematopoietic cells and 50 percent fat that is surrounded by bony trabeculae. The specific types of bone marrow cells can be difficult to recognize in histological sections at this low-power magnification, but the very large cells present are megakaryocytes. Cells are easier to identify on a smear from a bone marrow aspirate (Figure 1.3). The cells that are present include eryth-

rocytic and granulocytic precursors and a megakaryocyte. To classify these three different cell types, there are some general features that can be used. Megakaryocytes are easy to distinguish by their very large size; the majority of them are 100–200 μm in diameter compared with approximately 20–30 μm for the largest granulocytic or erythrocytic precursors.

Cells of the erythrocytic lineage can be initially distinguished from those of the granulocytic lineage on the basis of their nuclear shape and color of cytoplasm (Figs. 1.4 and 1.5). Cells of the erythrocytic lineage have very round nuclei throughout most stages of development. In contrast, the nuclei of cells of the granulocytic lineage become indented and segmented as they mature. In addition, the cytoplasm of early erythrocytic precursors is much bluer than that of the granulocytic precursors.

There are several additional common morphological features that occur during development of both erythrocytic and granulocytic precursors. Both cell and nucleus decrease in size as they mature. As cells lose their capacity to divide, there is a loss of nucleoli and a condensation of nuclear chromatin. Changes in the cytoplasm are also occurring. As the hemoglobin content in erythrocytic precursors increases, the cytoplasm becomes less blue and more red. As maturation proceeds in the granulocytic cells, the cytoplasm also becomes less blue.

Figure 1.2 Histological section of canine bone marrow. Pink bony trabeculae are present in the lower left corner, lower right corner, and top of the photomicrograph and surround the hematopoietic cells and fat. The round to oval clear areas are the fat. The erythrocytic and granulocytic precursor cells are the many small, round purple structures. The larger, densely staining purple structures distributed throughout the marrow space are megakaryocytes. Canine bone marrow core biopsy; hematoxylin and eosin stain; 10× objective.

Figure 1.3 Megakaryocyte, erythrocytic precursors, and granulocytic precursors. The megakaryocyte is the largest cell located in right center of the field. The early erythrocytic precursors have central round nuclei and deep blue cytoplasm. The early granulocytic precursors have oval to indented nuclei and blue cytoplasm. There is a granulocytic predominance in this field. Canine bone marrow smear; 50× objective.

Figure 1.4 Erythrocytic precursors. The majority of the intact cells present are early erythrocytic precursors with centrally located round nuclei and deep blue cytoplasm. The cells with round eccentrically placed nuclei and reddish-blue cytoplasm are late-stage erythrocytic precursors. The largest cell in the right center of the field that has small pink granules in the cytoplasm is a promyelocyte. Canine bone marrow smear; 100× objective.

Figure 1.5 Granulocytic precursors. The majority of the intact cells present are granulocytic precursors with oval to indented nuclei and blue cytoplasm. The larger immature forms have small, pink cytoplasmic granules. The cytoplasm becomes less blue as the cells mature. Canine bone marrow smear; 100× objective.

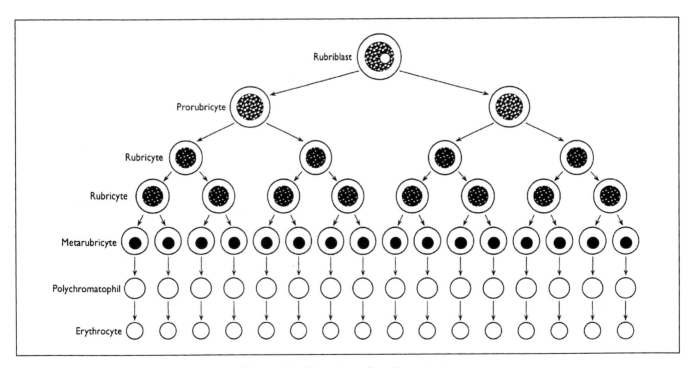

Figure 1.6 Overview of erythropoiesis.

ERYTHROPOIESIS

There are several stages of erythrocyte development that are recognizable in the bone marrow. Figure 1.6 depicts erythrocyte development, and Plate 1 (p. 10) shows the morphology of all erythrocytic precursors. Briefly, erythrocyte development is as follows.

The rubriblast is the first morphologically recognizable erythrocytic precursor. The rubriblast is a large, round cell with a large, round nucleus with coarsely granular chromatin and a prominent nucleolus. These cells have small amounts of deep blue cytoplasm. The rubriblast divides to produce two prorubricytes.

The prorubricyte is round and is of equal size or is sometimes larger than the rubriblast. The nucleus is round, with a coarsely granular chromatin pattern. A nucleolus is typically not present. There is a small amount of deep blue cytoplasm, often with a prominent perinuclear clear zone. Each prorubricyte divides to form two rubricytes.

The rubricyte is smaller than the prorubricyte. The nucleus is still round, and the coarsely granular chromatin is more condensed compared with the earlier stages. There is a small amount of deep blue cytoplasm, although some of the more mature rubricytes have reddish-blue cytoplasm. At the rubricyte stage, there are two divisions; the rubricytes then mature into metarubricytes.

The metarubricyte is smaller than the rubricyte. The nucleus is round to slightly oval, is centrally to eccentrically located, and has very condensed chromatin. There is a moderate amount of blue to reddish-blue cytoplasm. From the metarubricyte stage on, there is no further division of the cells, just maturation.

The highly condensed pyknotic nucleus of the metarubricyte is extruded from the cell, and this cell becomes a polychromatophil. Polychromatophils are round cells without a nucleus and have bluish cytoplasm. As a polychromatophil matures, it becomes less blue and more red, becoming a mature red blood cell. The mature red blood cells have species-depen-

dent morphological features, which are described in Chapter 2.

GRANULOPOIESIS

Granulopoiesis is depicted in Figure 1.7 and Plate 2 (p. 11). In the bone marrow, there are three types of granulocytes, which include cells of the neutrophilic, eosinophilic, and basophilic lineages. Cells of the neutrophilic lineage are the predominant type of granulocyte present, and their development is described first.

The myeloblast is the first recognizable granulocytic precursor in the bone marrow. It is a large cell with a round to oval nucleus with a finely granular chromatin pattern and one or more prominent nucleoli. The amount of cytoplasm is small to moderate and blue. Each myeloblast divides to form two promyelocytes. Promyelocytes look similar to myeloblasts except they may not have nucleoli, and they may have a perinuclear clear zone within the cytoplasm. The distinguishing feature of promyelocytes is that they contain multiple, very small, pink to purple granules in the cytoplasm; these are known as primary granules. Promyelocytes divide to produce myelocytes.

The myelocyte is smaller than the earlier precursors and has a round to oval to slightly indented nucleus with finely to moderately granular chromatin. These

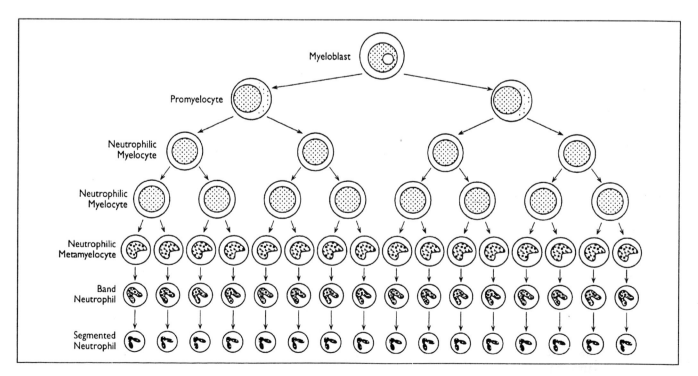

Figure 1.7 Overview of neutrophilic granulopoiesis.

cells have moderate amounts of blue cytoplasm. At this stage, primary granules are no longer being produced, and now secondary granules are formed. These secondary granules are larger than the primary granules.

In neutrophilic myelocytes, the secondary granules are light pink and are very difficult to recognize with the light microscope. The myelocyte goes through two divisions, and the resulting progeny mature into metamyelocytes. From the metamyelocyte stage forward, the cells no longer divide.

The metamyelocyte is smaller than the myelocyte and has a kidney-shaped nucleus. The chromatin is moderately granular and is more condensed and clumped than that in the myelocyte. The cytoplasm is blue and contains primary and secondary granules. Both types of granules in the metamyelocyte and subsequent stages of development are not easily seen light microscopically in most animal species. Metamyelocytes develop into band neutrophils. Band neutrophils are round and smaller than metamyelocytes, have horseshoe-shaped nuclei, and have moderate amounts of blue to light blue cytoplasm. The band neutrophil will mature into a segmented neutrophil, which is a small cell with faintly blue to pink cytoplasm and a segmented nucleus. The nuclear chromatin is coarsely granular and clumped.

Mature eosinophils and basophils and their precursors are found in very low numbers in the normal bone marrow. The production of these cells is very similar to that of neutrophils, and the only major differences are described in Figure 1.1. The development is identical until the myelocytic stage, which is when eosinophilic and basophilic myelocytes can be distinguished from neutrophilic myelocytes by the color of the secondary granules. The eosinophilic and basophilic myelocytes contain reddish to reddish-orange and purple secondary granules, respectively. Eosinophilic and basophilic metamyelocytes and bands can also be recognized by the presence of the unique secondary granules.

The last stage of development is the mature eosinophil and basophil. The eosinophil is often slightly larger than the mature neutrophil, and the nucleus is not as tightly segmented. The cytoplasm contains reddish to reddish-orange granules. The mature basophil is a round cell that is slightly larger than the neutrophil, with a segmented nucleus with condensed chromatin. The cytoplasm is light purple and may contain granules. There are some unique species-dependent features of mature eosinophils and basophils, which are described in Chapter 5.

MONOCYTOPOIESIS

The precursors of monocytes arise from committed stem cells, which are common precursors for both cells of the granulocytic and monocytic lineage. Monocyte development is depicted in Figure 1.1. In normal bone marrow, very few cells of the monocytic lineage are present. Monoblasts are the first microscopically recognizable precursors in bone marrow, although they can be impossible to differentiate from myeloblasts. Monoblasts give rise to promonocytes. A promonocyte is a large cell with an oval to sometimes indented nucleus with a reticular (netlike) or lacy chromatin pattern. These cells have small to moderate amounts of blue cytoplasm and can be difficult to distinguish from neutrophilic myelocytes or metamyelocytes. Promonocytes give rise to monocytes, which are larger than segmented neutrophils. The nucleus of the monocyte has multiple indentations. The nuclear chromatin has areas of condensation but has a lacy or reticular pattern compared with the condensed chromatin pattern of the mature neutrophil. The cytoplasm is moderate in amount and is typically blue-gray, often with discrete multiple vacuoles.

MEGAKARYOCYTOPOIESIS AND PLATELET PRODUCTION

Megakaryocytopoiesis is quite unique compared with the development of the other blood cells and is depicted in Figure 1.1. The megakaryoblasts are the first morphologically recognizable precursors of the megakaryocytic lineage in bone marrow but can be impossible to differentiate from other blast cells. The megakaryoblast is a large cell with a single round nucleus and prominent nucleolus. This cell differentiates into a promegakaryocyte, which is larger than the megakaryoblast and has a multilobed nucleus with dark blue agranular cytoplasm. The promegakaryocyte gives rise to the megakaryocyte (Figure 1.8), which is easily recognized in the bone marrow because of its large size (typically 100–200 μm). This large cell has a large, multilobulated nucleus and abundant granular cytoplasm.

Platelets are formed from the cytoplasm of megakaryocytes by the formation of a structure known as a proplatelet. The proplatelet is fragmented into multiple platelets. The resulting platelets are discoid-shaped small cells that do not have nuclei and that have light pink cytoplasm with sometimes distinct purple granules.

Figure 1.8 Megakaryocyte. The megakaryocyte is the large cell in the center with a multilobulated irregular nucleus and abundant granular cytoplasm. Canine bone marrow smear; 50× objective.

LYMPHOPOIESIS

Lymphocytes arise from the same common stem cell precursor as the other bone marrow cells (Fig. 1.1). Multiple stages of differentiation of lymphocytes in bone marrow cannot be recognized light microscopically, but there are two main types of lymphocytes that can be identified by immunophenotyping in the peripheral blood: B and T lymphocytes. These two cell types look similar and cannot be differentiated on the basis of morphology alone, but their functions are quite different. In bone marrow, low numbers of small lymphocytes and rarely seen medium and large lymphocytes are present (Fig. 1.9). The exact number of lymphocytes present in bone marrow is species dependent; however, rodents have a relatively greater abundance of bone marrow lymphocytes compared with the common domestic species.

The small lymphocyte is a small, round cell with a round to slightly indented nucleus. In some areas, the nuclear chromatin has a very smooth glassy appearance, and in other areas it is more clumped or smudged. Overall, the chromatin is not as condensed as that of a rubricyte, which is the cell type with which it is most often confused. The lymphocyte has a small amount of light blue cytoplasm. The medium and large lymphocytes, as the names imply, are larger than the small lymphocytes. The nuclei are round, and the chromatin is finely granular, with some areas of condensation. The nucleus of the large lymphocyte typically has a nucleolus and is known as a lymphoblast. Both cell types have small amounts of light to moderate blue cytoplasm.

Figure 1.9 Lymphocytes. The two smallest round cells (left center) that are slightly larger than red blood cells, with round to oval nuclei and small amounts of light blue cytoplasm, are small lymphocytes. The largest cell in the center is a neutrophilic granulocytic precursor. The round cell (above the granulocytic precursor) with a round nucleus, very condensed chromatin, and a rim of deep blue cytoplasm is a rubricyte. Feline bone marrow smear; 100× objective.

Figure 1.10 Plasma cells. The three cells (center) with eccentrically placed round nuclei; coarse, clumped chromatin; and a moderate amount of deep blue cytoplasm with perinuclear clear zones are plasma cells. The other cells are mainly granulocytic precursors. Canine bone marrow smear; 100× objective.

In addition to lymphocytes, low numbers of plasma cells can be seen in bone marrow (Fig. 1.10). These cells are the end stage of differentiation of B lymphocytes and are round with eccentrically placed round nuclei. The nuclear chromatin is very condensed and clumped, with clear areas between the clumps. Plasma cells have moderate amounts of deep blue cytoplasm with a prominent perinuclear clear zone.

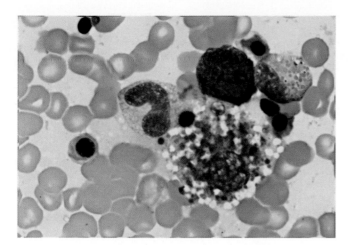

Figure 1.11 Macrophage. The large cell (right center) with abundant vacuolated cytoplasm and a round nucleus is a macrophage. The red-brown granules in the cytoplasm are consistent with hemosiderin. Canine bone marrow smear; 100× objective.

Figure 1.13 Osteoblasts. The nucleated cells with abundant blue cytoplasm (center) that form a circle are osteoblasts. These cells appear similar to plasma cells; however, they are larger than plasma cells, and the nuclear chromatin patterns are less coarse. Canine bone marrow smear; 100× objective.

Figure 1.12 Osteoclast. The very large cell (center) with multiple, individual round to oval nuclei and granular cytoplasm is an osteoclast. The large clear area in the lower right quadrant is a large fat droplet, which is partially indenting the osteoclast. Canine bone marrow smear; 50× objective.

OTHER CELLS OF THE BONE MARROW

Macrophage

Bone marrow macrophages are present in low numbers (Fig. 1.11). These cells are large and have an oval to indented nucleus. The nuclear chromatin is reticular (netlike). The moderate to abundant amounts of blue cytoplasm often are very foamy and may contain mul-

tiple, variably sized vacuoles. Often within these cells there can be phagocytized debris or iron pigment, known as hemosiderin. In general, hemosiderin is not identified in normal cat bone marrow but is readily identifiable in the marrow of most other common domestic and non-domestic species.

Osteoclast

Osteoclasts are rarely found in bone marrow smears. Osteoclasts are similar in size to megakaryocytes, and these two cell types are often confused (Fig. 1.12). The osteoclast has multiple, individual, round to oval nuclei. In contrast, the nucleus of the mature megakaryocyte is multilobulated. The osteoclast cytoplasm is granular and light blue to red.

Osteoblast

Osteoblasts are also found in very low numbers in normal bone marrow. The size of these cells is very similar to that of the macrophage, and the morphology is somewhat similar to that of the plasma cell, including an eccentrically placed round nucleus and prominent perinuclear clear zone (Fig. 1.13). The nucleus has a granular chromatin pattern, usually with a prominent single nucleolus. The cytoplasm is a light to moderate blue. In contrast, the plasma cell is smaller in size, and the nuclear chromatin is much more condensed, with no prominent nucleoli.

PLATE 1. Red Blood Cell Development

Rubriblast

The rubriblast is a large, round cell with a large, round nucleus; coarsely granular chromatin; and a nucleolus. This cell has small amounts of deep blue cytoplasm.

Prorubricyte

The prorubricyte is a large, round cell with a round nucleus with a coarsely granular chromatin pattern. This cell typically lacks a nucleolus. There is a small amount of deep blue cytoplasm often with a prominent perinuclear clear zone.

Rubricyte

The rubricyte is a round cell with a round, centrally located nucleus; it is smaller than the prorubricyte. The coarsely granular chromatin is more condensed compared with the earlier stages of development, and irregular clear areas are present between the chromatin clumps. The cytoplasm varies from deep blue to reddish-blue. Early rubricytes typically have more bluish cytoplasm, and later rubricytes stain more red as the amount of hemoglobin increases.

Metarubricyte

The metarubricyte is smaller than the rubricyte. The nucleus is round to oval, usually slightly eccentrically located, and has very condensed chromatin. There are small to moderate amounts of blue to reddish-blue cytoplasm. The metarubricytes, with more-reddish cytoplasm, contain more hemoglobin.

Polychromatophil

The polychromatophil does not have a nucleus, and cytoplasm is blue to reddish-blue. As polychromatophils mature, they become less blue and more red as a result of their increased amounts of hemoglobin.

Red Blood Cell

The red blood cell does not have a nucleus, and the cytoplasm is reddish to reddish-orange. The central pallor present here is a result of the biconcave discoid shape of the cells.

PLATE 2. White Blood Cell Development

Myeloblast

The myeloblast is a large, round to oval cell with a round to oval nucleus with a finely stippled chromatin pattern and usually prominent nucleolus or multiple nucleoli. There is a small to moderate amount of blue cytoplasm and no prominent cytoplasmic granules.

Promyelocyte

The promyelocyte is a large, round to oval cell with a round to oval nucleus. The nuclear chromatin pattern is finely granular. A nucleolus or multiple nucleoli may or may not be present. A perinuclear clear zone is often present but is not shown here. The moderate amount of cytoplasm is blue and contains multiple, fine, pink to purple granules, which are primary granules.

Neutrophilic Myelocyte

The neutrophilic myelocyte is a round cell that is smaller than the myeloblast and the progranulocyte. The nucleus is round to oval and may contain a single indentation. The chromatin pattern is finely to moderately granular. Nucleoli are not present. The moderate amounts of blue cytoplasm contain multiple secondary granules, also called specific granules. These secondary granules are pink for the neutrophilic lineage and are difficult to see. The secondary granules for the eosinophilic and basophilic lineages are generally reddish and purple, respectively.

Neutrophilic Metamyelocyte

The neutrophilic metamyelocyte is a round cell with a kidney-shaped nucleus. The chromatin is moderately granular and more condensed than that of the myelocyte. The moderate amounts of blue cytoplasm contain secondary granules, which are difficult to see. The secondary granules of the eosinophilic and basophilic metamyelocyte are generally reddish and purple, respectively.

Band Neutrophil

The band neutrophil is a round cell with a horseshoe-shaped nucleus. The nuclear membranes may have parallel sides, although slight indentations are acceptable. The cytoplasm is blue to light blue and contains secondary granules. These granules are difficult to see in the band neutrophil. The secondary granules of the band eosinophil and basophil are generally reddish and purple, respectively.

Segmented Neutrophil

The segmented neutrophil is a small round cell with a single nucleus, which has multiple segmentations. The nuclear chromatin is very condensed. There is a moderate amount of light blue to pink cytoplasm.

Figure 1.14 Mast cell. The cell (center) with abundant purple cytoplasmic granules is a mast cell. The granules almost obscure the round nucleus. A small fat droplet (round clear structure) is partially indenting the right side of the cell. Canine bone marrow smear; 100× objective.

Mast Cell

Mast cells are found in very low numbers in bone marrow in most species but can be found in higher numbers in the bone marrow of rats. These cells are round, with a round, centrally located nucleus (Fig. 1.14). These cells are easily recognized by the small purple granules that fill the cytoplasm. Often, in these cells the granularity is so great that it hides the nuclei. Mast cells are often present within intact bone marrow particles.

CHAPTER TWO
NORMAL RED BLOOD CELL MORPHOLOGY

The morphological features of mature red blood cells of most mammals are generally very similar in that they all lack nuclei, stain reddish to reddish-orange, and generally are biconcave, discoid-shaped cells. The major differences are found in the size of the red blood cells and the degree of central pallor. Listed from largest to smallest in size, common domestic species are dog, cat, horse, cow, sheep, and goat red blood cells. The central pallor is the lighter-staining area in the middle of the cell, resulting from a close association of the membranes in this region (Fig. 2.1). Dog red blood cells have the most prominent central pallor. In cats, horses, and ruminants, central pallor is not prominent. In contrast to the other domestic species, normal llama red blood cells are quite different in morphology. Although they lack nuclei and stain reddish to reddish-orange, they are small, elliptical discs that lack a biconcave shape and central pallor. Table 2.1 summarizes the morphological features, and Figures 2.2–2.8 show photomicrographs of normal red blood cells of the common domestic species. Figures 2.9–2.14 are photomicrographs of normal red blood cells of the nonhuman primate (cynomolgus monkey), rabbit (New Zealand White), guinea pig, ferret, rat (Sprague Dawley), and mouse (CD1). The size of the red blood cells in laboratory animals is dependent on the age of the animal that is being used, but in general, these species have red blood cell sizes that are of similar size or slightly smaller than dog red blood cells. In most laboratory animal species, the central pallor is not as pronounced as it is in the dog.

Two other morphological features that may be present in normal animals are rouleaux and anisocytosis. Rouleaux are organized linear arrays of red blood cells stacked one on top of another (see Fig. 3.8). This change can best be seen in thicker areas of blood smears, known as the body of the slide. Rouleaux are most prominent in normal horses, but they also occur in cats and, to a much lesser degree, in dogs. They are not commonly present in the normal state in common laboratory animal species. Rouleaux formation is related to differences in charges at the red blood cell surface, and changes in these charges can result in increased degrees of rouleaux formation. With inflam-

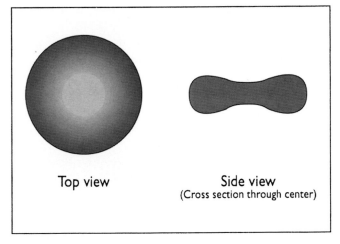

Top view   **Side view**
(Cross section through center)

Figure 2.1 Graphical representation of a normal dog red blood cell. Note that the central zone of pallor is a result of the closer apposition of membranes and a decreased amount of hemoglobin in this region.

Table 2.1
Morphological features of normal red blood cells

Animal	Diameter (μm)	Central Pallor	Rouleaux	Anisocytosis
Dog	7.0	++	+	−
Cat	5.8	+	++	+
Horse	5.7	±	+++	−
Cow	5.5	+	−	+
Sheep	4.5	+	±	±
Goat	3.2	±	±	+
Llama	4.0 × 7.0*	−	−	±

Source: Adapted from Jain, Nemi C. 1986. *Schalm's Veterinary Hematology*, 4th ed. Philadelphia: Lea & Febiger.

*Since these calls are not round, the approximate width and length of the cells are given.

matory disease, there often are increased levels of globulins in the blood that result in changes in surface charges, and thus increased rouleaux in most animals. In llamas and bovine species, there is generally a lack of rouleaux in normal and disease states. Anisocytosis is defined as a variation in red blood cell size. In the common domestic species, anisocytosis is mainly present in normal cats and cows (Figs. 2.3, 2.5). In the laboratory animal species, anisocytosis is present in the nonhuman primate, rabbit, ferret, guinea pig, mouse, and rat and is partially attributed to the higher numbers of polychromatophilic cells in some of these species, especially young animals.

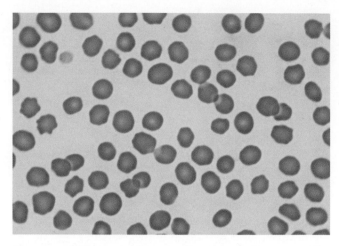

Figure 2.4 Horse red blood cells. These cells are smaller than dog red blood cells, and they have minimal central pallor. Equine blood smear; 100× objective.

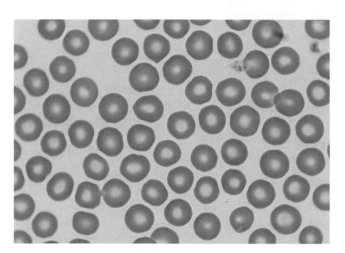

Figure 2.2 Dog red blood cells. The majority of the cells are of similar size and have prominent central pallor. Canine blood smear; 100× objective.

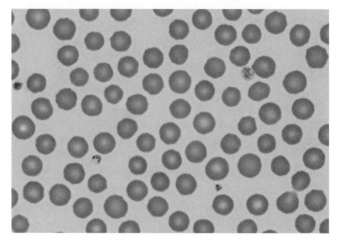

Figure 2.5 Cow red blood cells. There is slight variation in the size of these cells (anisocytosis), and they typically have limited central pallor. Bovine blood smear; 100× objective.

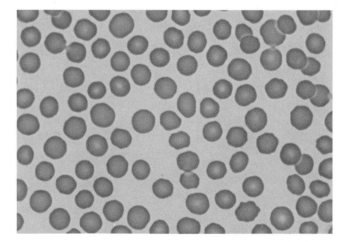

Figure 2.3 Cat red blood cells. These cells are smaller than dog red blood cells, there is slight variation in size (anisocytosis), and they have limited central pallor. Feline blood smear; 100× objective.

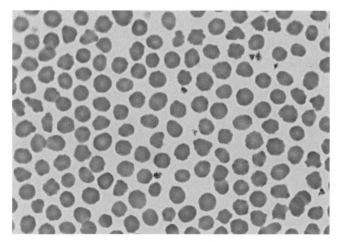

Figure 2.6 Sheep red blood cells. Note the very small size of these cells compared with dog red blood cells, as well as their limited central pallor. There is also a slight variation in the size (anisocytosis) and shape (poikilocytosis) of these cells. Ovine blood smear; 100× objective.

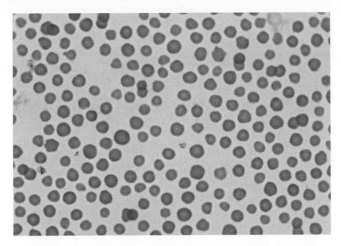

Figure 2.7 Goat red blood cells. Note the extremely small size of the cells and the minimal central pallor. It is also common to have a slight variation in size (anisocytosis) and shape (poikilocytosis). Caprine blood smear; 100× objective.

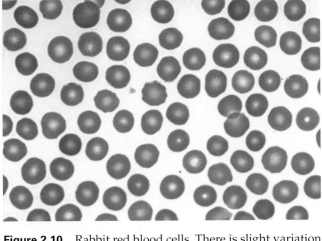

Figure 2.10 Rabbit red blood cells. There is slight variation in the size of the red blood cells (anisocytosis). The majority of the cells have a moderate amount of central pallor. Rabbit; 100× objective.

Figure 2.8 Llama red blood cells. These cells are elliptical and lack central pallor. Llama blood smear; 100× objective.

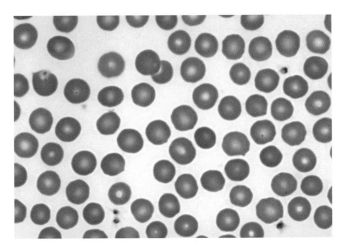

Figure 2.11 Guinea pig red blood cells. There is slight variation in the size of the red blood cells (anisocytosis). The majority of the cells have moderate amounts of central pallor. Guinea pig; 100× objective.

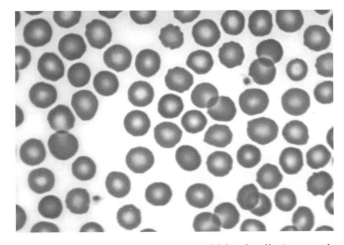

Figure 2.9 Nonhuman primate red blood cells (cynomolgus monkey). The majority of the cells have central pallor. There is slight variation in the size of the red blood cells. Nonhuman primate (cynomolgus monkey); 100× objective.

Figure 2.12 Ferret red blood cells. There is slight variation in the size of the red blood cells (anisocytosis). The majority of the cells have moderate amounts of central pallor. Ferret; 100× objective.

Figure 2.13 Mouse red blood cells. There is slight variation in the size of the red blood cells (anisocytosis). The majority of the cells have moderate amounts of central pallor. The bluish cell in the center of the field is a polychromatophil. Mouse; 100× objective.

Figure 2.14 Rat red blood cells. There is slight variation in the size of the red blood cells (anisocytosis). The majority of the cells have moderate amounts of central pallor. The two bluish cells in the center of the field with prominent central pallor are polychromatophils. Rat; 100× objective.

CHAPTER THREE

VARIATIONS IN RED BLOOD CELL MORPHOLOGY

Variations in the morphology of red blood cells can occur in animals with various disease and pathophysiological states. To better understand the development of these changes, they are grouped into five categories of morphological features: those associated with a regenerative response, immune-mediated damage, oxidative injury, membrane/metabolic disorder, and mechanical fragmentation. These categories are not mutually exclusive, and morphological features that are described in one category may be seen in multiple physiological or disease states. The more common physiological or disease states in which these cell types are seen are mentioned, but these lists are not meant to be comprehensive. These changes will often be demonstrated by photomicrographs of canine blood smears, but most of these abnormalities occur in the other species as well.

A general term that is used in describing variations in red blood cell morphology is "poikilocytosis," which is defined as abnormally shaped red blood cells in circulation. If the shape change that is present can be subclassified using a more specific term, the more specific term should be used.

REGENERATIVE RESPONSE

Anemias can be classified into two major categories: nonregenerative and regenerative. A nonregenerative anemia is the result of inadequate production of red blood cells by bone marrow; red blood cells that are present in circulation often appear normal. In contrast, a regenerative anemia is one in which the bone marrow has responded to a demand for red blood cells by increasing production and releasing into the circulation adequate numbers of immature red blood cells, known as polychromatophils (Fig. 3.1). These cells are also present in low numbers in the normal state in most of the common domestic species. In most of the common laboratory animal species, especially rats, polychromatophilic cells are present in higher numbers as a result of the shorter red blood cell lifespan and the younger age at which these animals are used. Polychromatophilic cells have bluish to reddish-blue cytoplasms and are typically slightly larger than mature

red blood cells. Also, because of the increased pliability of these cells, they do not always take on the classic discoid shape but may have multiple infoldings or outfoldings of the membranes and thus appear as target or bar cells, which are described next. Although polychromatophils can be identified on Wright's-stained preparations because of their bluish coloration, they can also be identified easily as reticulocytes by staining a blood sample with new methylene blue.

In new methylene blue–stained preparations, polychromatophils are called reticulocytes (Fig. 3.2), and they stain bluish-green, as do mature red blood cells. In addition, the polychromatophils will have irregular netlike structures, known as reticulum, within the cells. The reticulum is irregular clumps of ribosomal RNA and organelles, such as mitochondria. In most species, there is only one type of reticulocyte. However, in cats there are two forms of reticulocytes: punctate and aggregate (Fig. 3.3). The aggregate reticulocytes have abundant reticulum, whereas punctate reticulocytes have only a few isolated dots of reticulum, which do not coalesce.

In addition to finding polychromatophils, other features that may be seen in regenerative anemias are nucleated red blood cells, basophilic stippling, anisocytosis, and Howell-Jolly bodies. It is not exactly clear why nucleated red blood cells (Fig. 3.4) are found in circulation during a regenerative response. It may be that these cells are released as a result of mild bone marrow stromal damage, because of the increased demand for red blood cells, or extramedullary hematopoiesis.

When demand for red blood cells is great, production occurs in extramedullary sites such as the liver and spleen, with the subsequent potential release of nucleated red blood cells into circulation. When nucleated red blood cells are present without the presence of adequate polychromasia, underlying causes of bone marrow damage are likely. A classic example of this is seen in animals with lead poisoning or with marrow infiltrative disease (primary and metastatic neoplasia).

Basophilic stippling (Fig. 3.5) can be seen on Wright's-stained smears as small, variably sized blue dots in the cytoplasm of red blood cells. In most cases,

Figure 3.1 Polychromatophils. The bluish-staining, usually larger red blood cells are polychromatophils. In most animals except horses, polychromatophils are present in high numbers in circulation during a regenerative anemia. In addition, there is slight poikilocytosis, and target cells are present. Canine blood smear; 100× objective.

Figure 3.3 Aggregate and punctate reticulocytes. The two cells (left center) that have dark blue, clumped granular material in the cytoplasm are aggregate reticulocytes. The cells with small single or multiple dots of bluish material are punctate reticulocytes. The cells with no reticulum are mature red blood cells. Feline blood smear; new methylene blue stain; 100× objective.

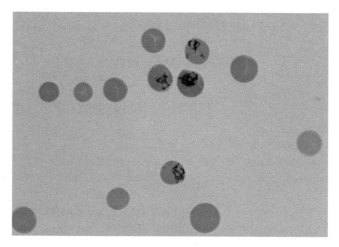

Figure 3.2 Reticulocytes. The four cells with dark blue, clumped granular material (reticulum) in the cytoplasm are reticulocytes. The cells with no reticulum are mature red blood cells. Canine blood smear; new methylene blue stain; 100× objective.

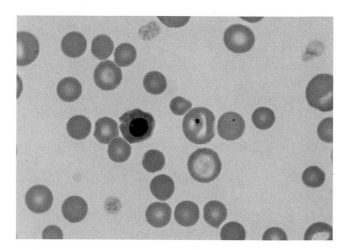

Figure 3.4 Nucleated red blood cell and Howell-Jolly bodies. The slightly blue cell with the round nucleus and condensed chromatin is a nucleated red blood cell (metarubricyte). Two adjacent red blood cells have single, small, round, deep purple cytoplasmic inclusions; these are Howell-Jolly bodies, which are fragments of nuclei. Canine blood smear; 100× objective.

the dots are retained RNA and are most commonly seen during regenerative responses in ruminants, but they also can be seen during regeneration in other species. Basophilic stippling may be seen in lead poisoning because lead inhibits an enzyme that is important in the degradation of RNA.

Anisocytosis has been previously defined and occurs in a regenerative response, typically resulting from the presence of large polychromatophils.

Howell-Jolly bodies (Fig. 3.4) are remnant fragments of nuclear material present in red blood cells. Their

presence during a regenerative response is probably the result of the inability of macrophages to fully remove the nuclei of the maturing red blood cells during accelerated production. If Howell-Jolly bodies are present with a lack of adequate polychromasia, then decreased macrophagic function should be considered, especially splenic macrophagic function. A normal animal that has been splenectomized will often have Howell-Jolly bodies in circulation.

Figure 3.5 Basophilic stippling. The red blood cell (center) with multiple, small blue dots is a red blood cell with basophilic stippling. The three large, bluish-staining red blood cells are polychromatophils. There also is moderate anisocytosis present. Bovine blood smear; 100× objective.

Figure 3.7 Agglutination. There are several irregular clusters of red blood cells present; this is agglutination. These are present throughout the field, but three large clumps are present (center). Agglutination may be seen in animals with immune-mediated anemia. Equine blood smear; 50× objective.

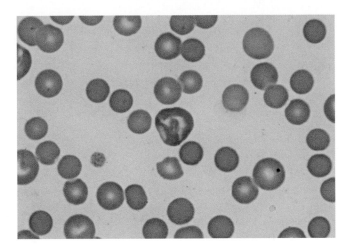

Figure 3.6 Spherocytes. The smaller cells that lack central pallor are spherocytes. These cells may be present in relatively high numbers in animals with immune-mediated hemolytic anemia. There is also a polychromatophil (center) and a red blood cell (lower right) with a Howell-Jolly body. Canine blood smear; 100× objective.

Figure 3.8 Rouleaux. The linear and sometimes branching chains of red blood cells is rouleaux formation. Under normal conditions, this finding is most prominent in horses; however, rouleaux may be seen in increased amounts associated with inflammatory disease in most species. Equine blood smear; 50× objective.

IMMUNE-MEDIATED DAMAGE

Red blood cell morphological abnormalities associated with erythrocytic-directed immune-mediated processes result in the possibility of finding spherocytes, agglutination, and ghost cells. Spherocytes (Fig. 3.6) are formed by macrophages partially removing antibody-coated membranes. Because of the membrane loss, these cells can no longer retain their normal discoid shape, and thus a spherical shape with a lack of central pallor is produced. These cells are most easily recognized in dogs and other species with prominent central pallor. Spherocytes may be present in low numbers when there is nonimmune-mediated damage to the red blood cells as well.

Agglutination (Fig. 3.7) is an unorganized three-dimensional clustering of red blood cells, typically formed as a result of a cross-linking of red blood cell surface–associated antibodies. Agglutination also has been seen in horses that were treated with heparin. Agglutination may be seen both macroscopically and microscopically and must be distinguished from rouleaux formation (Fig. 3.8), which is related to the charges on red blood cells.

Figure 3.9 Ghost cells. The four very pale, small red blood cells are ghost cells. These indicate intravascular hemolysis. Also visible are spherocytes, polychromatophils, and a red blood cell with a large Howell-Jolly body. Canine blood smear; 100× objective.

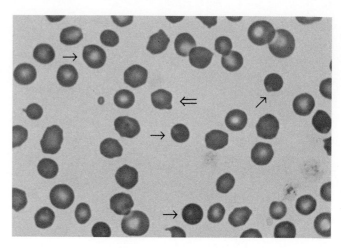

Figure 3.11 Heinz bodies. The red blood cell (double arrow) has a small round projection from the surface at the five o'clock position that is a Heinz body. Many of the red blood cells also have small, round, clear structures on their surface (single arrows) that are also Heinz bodies. Feline blood smear; 100× objective.

Figure 3.10 Heinz bodies. The small round projections from the surface of the red blood cells (center) are Heinz bodies. These represent oxidation and denaturation of hemoglobin. Canine blood smear; 100× objective.

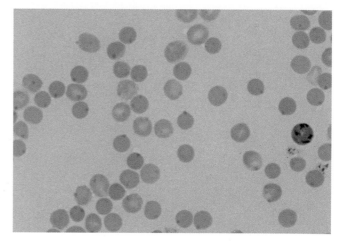

Figure 3.12 Heinz bodies. The red blood cell (center) has a Heinz body, which is the small, round, light blue-green projection from the surface at the twelve o'clock position. Many of the red blood cells throughout the field also have single, or sometimes multiple, Heinz bodies. There is also an aggregate reticulocyte (right center). Feline blood smear; new methylene blue stain; 100× objective.

Ghost cells (Fig. 3.9) are remnant membranes of red blood cells that have undergone intravascular lysis. This lysis can be induced by binding antibody and complement to the red blood cell membrane as well as other non–immune mediated mechanisms.

OXIDATIVE INJURY

Oxidation of red blood cells may occur during some disease states, as well as with exposure to certain drugs. This oxidation and denaturation of hemoglobin in red blood cells results in the formation of protuberances from the red blood cell membrane that are often

refractile; these are known as Heinz bodies (Figs. 3.10 and 3.11). If the Heinz bodies are large, they can easily be seen on Wright's-stained smears. These structures can also be identified using new methylene blue–stained smears, in which they stain light greenish-blue (Fig. 3.12). Heinz bodies are often seen more commonly in cats.

Another cell type that is sometimes present on exposure to oxidants is the eccentrocyte (Fig. 3.13). These cells have crescent-shaped clear areas that are

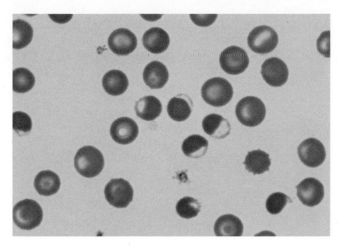

Figure 3.13 Eccentrocytes. The four red blood cells (center) with peripheral clear areas and displaced hemoglobin are eccentrocytes. Others are located at the periphery of the field. These represent oxidation of red blood cell membranes. Canine blood smear; 100× objective.

Figure 3.14 Echinocytes. The majority of the red blood cells have small uniform spines projecting from the surface. These are echinocytes. The most common cause of echinocyte formation is an in vitro artifact, known as crenation. Canine blood smear; 100× objective.

eccentrically placed. This clear area represents where cell membranes are closely apposed and possibly bonded as a result of oxidant-induced membrane damage.

Metabolic/Membrane Disorders

The exposure of red blood cells to different environments, both in vitro and in vivo, can result in morphological variations from the normal discoid shape. One of the more common variations seen is the echinocyte. Echinocytes are cells with multiple, small, delicate, regular-shaped spines distributed evenly around red blood cell membranes. The most common cause of echinocyte formation is an in vitro artifact, crenation (Figs. 3.14 and 3.15), which morphologically can be difficult to distinguish from true echinocytes. Of all the common laboratory animal species, rat (Sprague Dawley) red blood cells easily crenate. True echinocytes occur in association with different metabolic disorders such as renal disease. Collecting and immediately fixing blood before exposure to glass or an anticoagulant is required to distinguish true echinocytes from crenation.

Burr cells (Fig. 3.16) have multiple projections similar to echinocytes but are oval to elongate. Burr cells may be seen in animals with renal disease. The burr cell term is also sometimes used as a synonym for crenation in human hematology.

Figure 3.15 Echinocytes. The majority of the red blood cells have small spines projecting from the surface. These are echinocytes. The most common cause of echinocyte formation is an in vitro artifact, known as crenation. Rat blood smear; 100× objective.

In contrast to echinocytes, acanthocytes (Fig. 3.17) are cells with multiple (two to ten), irregularly shaped, blunt, finger-like projections. These cells are formed as a result of alterations in the ratio of cholesterol and phospholipids in the red blood cell membranes. Acanthocytes are commonly seen in animals with liver disease and are often found in dogs with hemangiosarcoma; they may be caused by the neoplastic involvement of the liver or by an unusual fragmentation resulting from the tortuosity of the neoplastic vasculature. Acanthocytes may also potentially be seen in association with renal disease–induced lipid abnormalities.

Figure 3.16 Burr cells. The elongated red blood cells with multiple, short blunt projections from the surface are burr cells. These cells may be seen in animals with renal disease. Feline blood smear; 100× objective.

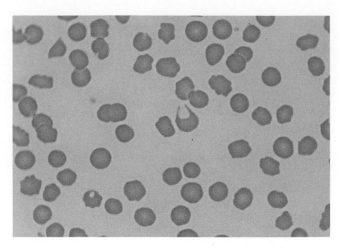

Figure 3.18 Keratocyte. The cell with two hornlike projections (center) is a keratocyte. Feline blood smear; 100× objective.

Figure 3.17 Acanthocytes. Note the red blood cells with multiple irregularly shaped projections from the surface. This abnormality is associated with alterations in cholesterol and phospholipid ratios in the membrane. These cells may be seen in animals with liver disease. Canine blood smear; 100× objective.

Figure 3.19 Blister cell. The cell with a thin piece of membrane extending from the surface (center) is a blister cell. This blister often ruptures to form a keratocyte. Hypochromic cells are also present. Canine blood smear; 100× objective.

Keratocytes (Fig. 3.18) are cells with two fairly uniform hornlike projections. These are thought to arise from a localized area of membrane damage in which a vacuole or blister is formed in the red blood cell membrane and that subsequently ruptures. The cells with intact blister-like membrane structures are commonly known as blister cells (Fig. 3.19).

There are several potentially significant morphological changes associated with the zone of central pallor. These changes include hypochromasia, stomatocytosis, ovalocytosis, and leptocytosis. Two cell types that have an accentuation of the central pallor

are hypochromic cells and torocytes. In hypochromic cells (Figs. 3.20 and 3.21), there is increased central pallor, and the cells stain a lighter red as a result of their having a decreased amount of hemoglobin. As with normal red blood cells, there is a gradual transition between the outer and more dense staining regions of the cells and the central zone of pallor. Hypochromic cells are present in animals with iron deficiency because iron is needed for normal hemoglobin synthesis. In contrast, in torocytes (Fig. 3.22), although there is accentuated central pallor, the diameter of the central pallor region is not typically as great

Figure 3.20 Hypochromic cells. There are several hypochromic cells throughout the field that have pronounced central pallor as well as faintly staining cell membranes. This change is most often associated with iron deficiency. Canine blood smear; 100× objective.

Figure 3.22 Torocyte. The majority of the cells in the field are torocytes, commonly known as punched-out cells. These cells have prominent central pallor with an abrupt transition from the pale center to the outer portion of the cell. They also may appear as smaller-than-normal red blood cells. The torocyte morphology is typically an artifact resulting from abnormal spreading of cells on the slide. Canine blood smear; 100× objective.

Figure 3.21 Hypochromic cells. The majority of the cells that have central pallor are hypochromic cells. A few normal llama red blood cells that typically lack central pallor are also present. This change is most often associated with iron deficiency. The fusiform shape of some of the cells is an additional common feature in llamas with iron deficiency. Llama blood smear; 100× objective.

Figure 3.23 Stomatocyte. The somewhat oval cell with a linear central pallor (center) is a stomatocyte. Many target cells are also present. Canine blood smear; 100× objective.

as that of hypochromic cells, the overall density of the red coloration of the cell is normal, and there is an abrupt transition between the outer and central zones of the cell. Torocytes are also commonly known as punched-out cells and are usually artifacts of preparation.

Stomatocytes (Fig. 3.23) are cells in which the central pallor is more oval to elongate and takes on the appearance of a mouth. If these cells are evaluated in wet mount preparations, they are seen as being folded over on themselves in one direction. Stomatocytes have been seen in animals with red blood cell inherited metabolic or acquired membrane defects, but they also can be found as an artifact of preparation in the thicker areas of the slide.

Ovalocytes (Fig. 3.24), also known as elliptocytes, are cells that are oval, with an oval region of central pallor. They have been seen in animals with red blood cell membrane defects. They are normal in llamas.

Leptocytes are cells that are larger than normal mature red blood cells and have excessively thin

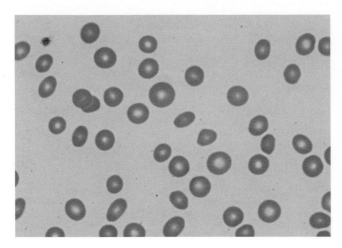

Figure 3.24 Ovalocytes. The oval red blood cells present are ovalocytes. They may be seen in animals with red blood cell membrane defects. Feline blood smear; 100× objective.

Figure 3.26 Bar cell. The cell (center) with a bar-shaped portion of membrane bisecting the area of central pallor is a bar cell, also known as a knizocyte. The change represents an outfolding of the red blood cell membrane similar to the change in the many target cells in this field. Canine blood smear; 100× objective.

Figure 3.25 Target cells. Many of the red blood cells with a target-like appearance are target cells, also known as codocytes. The central area of the cells that stains represents an outfolding of the red blood cell membrane in this region. These cells may be found in animals with liver disease or with polychromasia. Canine blood smear; 100× objective.

Figure 3.27 Schistocytes. The irregularly shaped red blood cell (center) is a schistocyte, or red blood cell fragment. There are two very small schistocytes in the lower right quadrant. Two larger fragments are present (upper left). This change is related to mechanical damage to the red blood cell. Canine blood smear; 100× objective.

membranes that tend to fold easily. Two types of leptocytes include target cells and bar cells.

Target cells (Fig. 3.25), also known as codocytes, have an extra, round outfolding of the membrane in the middle of the cell that gives the cell a target-like appearance. Because polychromatophils often are very pliable, it is common for them to take on the appearance of a target cell. Target cell morphology is somewhat of a nonspecific change, but if it occurs in high numbers of mature red blood cells, investigation into possible liver disease should be considered.

Bar cells (Fig. 3.26), also known as knizocytes, have a central, bar-shaped outfolding of the membrane. Bar

cells are often seen in similar situations as target cells.

MECHANICAL FRAGMENTATION

Schistocytes (Fig. 3.27), also known as schizocytes, are fragments of red blood cells. These fragments result from mechanical damage to red blood cells in circula-

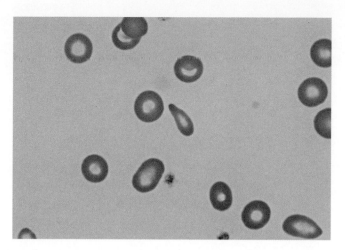

Figure 3.28 Dacryocyte. The teardrop-shaped red blood cell (center) is a dacryocyte. These cells may be seen in animals with myelofibrosis. Canine blood smear; 100× objective.

tion, often caused by microvascular abnormalities. One of the more common abnormalities that leads to schistocyte formation is the presence of fibrin strands in the microvasculature. These strands can cut red blood cells into two or more irregularly shaped pieces as the cells traverse the vasculature. A common pathophysiological state in which these changes may be seen is disseminated intravascular coagulation.

Dacryocytes (Fig. 3.28) are teardrop-shaped red blood cells. It is not exactly clear how these cells are formed, but this change may represent a type of fragmentation. Dacryocytes may be seen in animals with myelofibrosis.

CHAPTER FOUR
RED BLOOD CELL
INCLUSIONS AND PARASITES

In evaluating red blood cells for inclusions or parasites, there are several normal structures and artifacts that often confuse the novice hematologist. Some of these structures were defined in Chapter 3 but are reviewed here briefly. In addition, for many red blood cell parasites, there are now polymerase chain reaction–based tests that can be used to help identify the organisms. One of the most common artifacts that is confused with red blood cell parasites or inclusions is stain precipitate (Fig. 4.1), which presents as small, variably sized, pink to purple granular material. It often can be found on red blood cells as well as in the background of the slide; it is generally in a different plane of focus than the red blood cells. This distribution and size variability is helpful in distinguishing stain precipitate from true red blood cell parasites. In contrast, basophilic stippling (retained RNA aggregates; Fig. 4.2) appears as very small, multiple, round blue granules in the cytoplasm of the red blood cell. As previously stated in Chapter 3, this material is generally retained aggregates of RNA in the cell. Basophilic stippling is difficult to distinguish from Pappenheimer bodies, which are small blue granules in red blood cells. Pappenheimer bodies are aggregates of iron accumulation in the red blood cells (Fig. 4.3). Anucleated and nucleated red blood cells with Pappenheimer bodies are known as siderocytes and sideroblasts, respectively. A special stain, such as a Prussian blue, is the only way to confirm the presence of Pappenheimer bodies. When small blue granules are present in the red blood cells, they are most likely basophilic stippling, not Pappenheimer bodies.

Another artifact that may be confused with erythrocytic parasites is red blood cell refractile artifacts (Fig. 4.4). It is not clear how these form. This material can take on several sizes and shapes but can be confused with erythrocytic parasites when it is of similar size to such organisms as *Mycoplasma* spp, formerly known as *Haemobartonella*. The main feature used to distinguish this artifact from a true parasite is that these structures are variably sized and refractile when the microscope is focused up and down.

Finally, on occasion, platelets may be seen on top of red blood cells and thus appear to be inclusions (Fig. 4.5). By comparing the platelet on top of the red blood cell with those platelets present throughout the rest of the slide, it should be distinguishable from true red cell inclusions or parasites.

Figure 4.1 Stain precipitate. The variably sized, purple granular material present on and between the red blood cells is stain precipitate. Canine blood smear; 100× objective.

Figure 4.2 Basophilic stippling. Several of the red blood cells have very small, variably sized, pale blue granules, which are known as basophilic stippling. This is best demonstrated in the two red blood cells in the lower left quadrant. A metarubricyte is present in the upper right quadrant. Canine blood smear; 100× objective.

Figure 4.3 Pappenheimer bodies. The very small, poorly distinct, pale blue granules found in some of the red blood cells are Pappenheimer bodies. These are best demonstrated in the three red blood cells that are in a row in the lower right quadrant. These inclusions are a result of iron accumulation. In contrast, the red blood cell in the center of the field contains a small, round, deep purple structure, which is a Howell-Jolly body. Canine blood smear, from 1988 American Society for Veterinary Clinical Pathology slide review, courtesy of J. A. Matthews; 100× objective.

Figure 4.4 Refractile artifact. The round to oval—or irregularly shaped and variably sized—shiny unstained structures present on the surface of the red blood cells are refractile artifacts. Bovine blood smear; 100× objective.

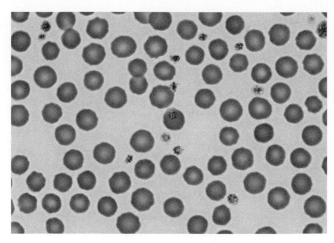

Figure 4.5 Erythrocyte pseudoinclusion. A platelet superimposed on a red blood cell is present in the center of the field. Note the similar features to the other platelets. Bovine blood smear; 100× objective.

Figure 4.6 Howell-Jolly bodies. Four red blood cells have single, small, round, deep purple cytoplasmic inclusions; these are Howell-Jolly bodies, which are nuclear fragments. Target cells are also present. Canine blood smear; 100× objective.

Howell-Jolly bodies (Fig. 4.6) are remnant micronuclei that may be seen in most domestic species during a regenerative anemia. These structures stain dark purple and are approximately 1 μm in diameter, although they can be larger. A single micronucleus typically is present in a red blood cell. In ruminants, *Anaplasma* organisms (Fig. 4.7) can look very similar in size, shape, and staining intensity to Howell-Jolly bodies. Fortunately, the most common type of ana-plasmosis is a result of *Anaplasma marginale*, which, as the name implies, is often found at the periphery of the red blood cell. Although Howell-Jolly bodies can be found on the edge of the cell, the majority of these structures are more randomly distributed in the red blood cells. In addition, in anaplasmosis, more than one organism per cell is often present, whereas with Howell-Jolly bodies, the micronuclei are usually single. Because anaplasmosis often causes a regenerative anemia, both *Anaplasma* and Howell-Jolly bodies may be present concurrently.

Viral inclusions can be found in red blood cells (Fig. 4.8) and white blood cells in dogs with acute distem-

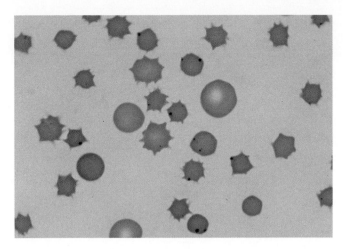

Figure 4.7 *Anaplasma marginale.* The single to multiple, round, deep purple cytoplasmic inclusions in several of the red blood cells are *A. marginale* organisms. Note that many of these organisms are present on the extreme periphery of the red blood cell. Bovine blood smear; 100× objective.

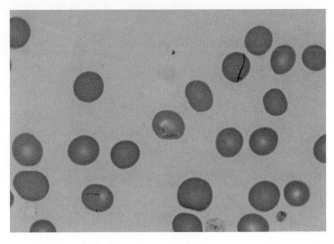

Figure 4.9 *Mycoplasma haemocanis.* The very small, coccoid- to rod-shaped blue structures forming chains on several of the red blood cells are *M. haemocanis* organisms. Canine blood smear; 100× objective.

Figure 4.8 Distemper viral inclusions. The variably sized, round, reddish-pink structures present in five of the red blood cells are canine distemper viral inclusions. Canine blood smear; 100× objective.

Figure 4.10 *Babesia canis.* There are two *B. canis* organisms within the red blood cell in the middle of the field. These are light blue pyriform structures with internal purple bodies. Inset (upper right) is a greater magnification of the organisms. Canine blood smear; Diff-Quik stain; 100× objective.

per virus infection. These inclusions are quite variable in size but usually are much larger than Howell-Jolly bodies. Viral inclusions can be several microns in diameter and are round to oblong to quite variably shaped. They typically stain pink to red, although more-bluish inclusions have been reported. Generally, there is no real internal structure, and often the inclusion has a smooth glassy appearance, although it may be granular. Diff-Quik stain is often stated as the preferred stain for identifying viral inclusions.

The common red blood cell parasites of dogs are *Mycoplasma haemocanis*, formerly *Haemobartonella canis*, and *Babesia sp. (B. canis* and *B. gibsoni). M. haemocanis*

(Fig. 4.9) is a very small epicellular parasite, less than 1 μm in diameter, and may be difficult to distinguish from stain artifact. It is coccoid or rod shaped and can be found individually or in groups on red blood cells. The organism often forms chains across the red blood cells. Babesiosis is most commonly caused by *B. canis* (Fig. 4.10) and is found mainly in the southeastern United States, South and Central America, Southern Europe, Africa, Asia, and Australia. This large, intracellular, pyriform-shaped parasite is easy to recognize, although often very few cells in a blood smear contain organisms. These organisms are typically 2.5–

3 μm wide by 4–5 μm long. Multiple organisms may be present in the cell. *B. gibsoni* (Fig. 4.11; United States, Southern Europe, Asia) also causes disease in dogs and is typically a much smaller, round to oval to elongate organism.

The most common red blood cell parasite of cats is *Mycoplasma* spp, formerly known as *Haemobartonella* spp. and has a worldwide distribution. *Mycoplasma haemofelis*, formerly *Haemobartonella felis* (Fig. 4.12), is a small, coccoid- to rod-shaped epicellular organism similar in morphology to *M. haemocanis*. This

Figure 4.11 *Babesia gibsoni.* Single to multiple *B. gibsoni* organisms are located within several red blood cells. Inset (upper left) is a greater magnification demonstrating pale blue ring forms with pinpoint purple bodies. Canine blood smear; 100× objective.

Mycoplasma has also been referred to as the Ohio organism, or large form. In addition, ring forms also may be seen. As with *M. haemocanis*, *M. haemofelis* can be difficult to distinguish from stain precipitate. Another type of *Mycoplasma* has also been recognized in cats; the proposed name for it is *Mycoplasma haemominutum* and it has a similar morphology to *M. haemofelis*. It has also been called the California organism, or small form. It requires a good-quality, well-stained blood smear for accurate identification of all the feline *Mycoplasma*. Attachment of the organisms to the outside of the cell is not very strong, and thus the organisms can be removed easily. If there is a delay in making an air-dried blood smear from EDTA anticoagulated blood, organisms may be found in the background of the slide and not on the red blood cells.

Cytauxzoon felis (Fig. 4.13) is another red blood cell parasite of cats. It is often bluish-staining and oval (1–5 μm in diameter) with a clear central region. Often a purple nucleus is on one end of the oval, giving the organism a signet ring appearance. Some organisms have chromatin bodies on both ends, giving them a "safety pin" appearance. Typically, these organisms are present in the blood in low numbers. Most cases have been reported in Missouri and the rest of the southern United States, southern Europe, Africa, and South and Central America.

In ruminants, *Anaplasma* (United States, subtropical and tropical areas) and *Babesia* (worldwide distribution, with the exception of the United States) are

Figure 4.12 *Mycoplasma haemofelis.* Many of the red blood cells have single or multiple; small; blue; coccoid-, rod-, or ring-shaped organisms on their surface. These organisms are *M. haemofelis*. Inset (upper left) is a greater magnification of these organisms. Feline blood smear; 100× objective.

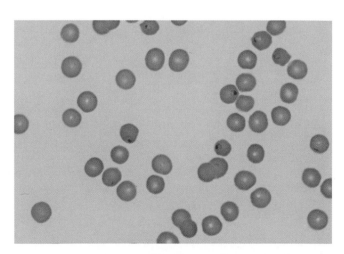

Figure 4.13 *Cytauxzoon felis.* Three red blood cells in the center of the field have blue rings, each with a single, eccentrically located purple nucleus. These organisms are *C. felis*. Feline blood smear; 100× objective.

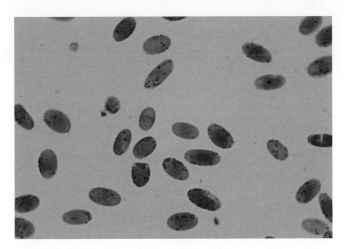

Figure 4.14 *Mycoplasma haemolamae.* The single or multiple; small; blue coccoid-, rod-, or ring-shaped organisms on the surface of these red blood cells are *Mycoplasma haemolamae.* Llama blood smear; 100× objective.

the most common red blood cell parasites. In cattle, anaplasmosis is most often caused by *A. marginale* (Fig. 4.7). These organisms are approximately 1 μm in diameter, are coccoid shaped, stain dark purple, and are often located on the periphery of the red blood cells; one to a few organisms may be present per red blood cell. As stated earlier, these organisms must be distinguished from Howell-Jolly bodies. In an infected animal, many red blood cells usually contain the parasite.

Another parasite of ruminants, as well as of llamas, is *Eperythrozoon* (Fig. 4.14). Recently, these species have been reclassified and renamed *Mycoplasma* spp. *Mycoplasma wenyonii,* formerly *Eperythrozoon wenyoni* (worldwide distribution), is the organism that typically infects cattle; *Mycoplasma ovis,* formerly *Eperythrozoon ovis,* affects sheep worldwide. In llamas, the exact species of the organism has not been determined, although recently the name *Mycoplasma haemolamae* has been proposed. In both ruminants and llamas, the organisms look very similar to *M. haemofelis.* These organisms can appear as coccoid-, rod-, or ring-shaped structures on the surface of the red blood cell. They are approximately 0.5 μm in diameter. Multiple organisms are often found on red blood cells, and organisms may be found in the background of the slide as well.

NORMAL WHITE BLOOD CELL MORPHOLOGY

SEGMENTED NEUTROPHIL

Segmented neutrophils are the most common white blood cells found in the peripheral blood of all the common domestic species, except ruminants, where lymphocytes are the predominant white blood cell. Similar to ruminants, in most laboratory animal species, the percentage of lymphocytes is often greater than the neutrophils. Segmented neutrophils are typically 10–12 μm in diameter and have single nuclei with several indentations, resulting in the nucleus being divided into multiple lobes. Typically there are three to five lobes or segments per cell. Neutrophils from normal nonhuman primates, such as the cynomolgus monkey, will often have up to eight segments per cell. The chromatin pattern of the nucleus consists of very dark, condensed areas intermixed with small, clear areas. The cytoplasm stains faintly blue to pink depending on the type and quality of the stain used. Sometimes very indistinct pink granules may be seen in the cytoplasm. The neutrophils of the different common domestic species look very similar. The major exception is that the cytoplasm of bovine neutrophils often stains pinker compared with that of the other species. Also, in horses, the segments of the nucleus are generally not as distinct. In the common laboratory animal species, the neutrophil is similar in size and shape to the common domestic species, but they often have prominent small cytoplasmic granules of varying numbers. The granules are smaller than the granules present in the eosinophil, and thus these cells can be easily distinguished. The rabbit and guinea pig have especially prominent granules, and thus these cells have been called pseudoeosinophils. In the rabbit, the proper term for these cells is "heterophils." Neutrophils in normal mice and rats may have ring-shaped nuclei.

BAND NEUTROPHIL

Band neutrophils may be absent or present in the peripheral blood in very low numbers. Band neutrophils look similar to segmented neutrophils except that the nuclei are band shaped. Classically, the nuclear membranes are parallel so that the nucleus has a constant width. Because band neutrophils are a stage in the gradual differentiation toward the segmented-neutrophil form, slight nuclear indentations are possible. Cytoplasmic granules of varying numbers may be present in most of the common laboratory animal species.

LYMPHOCYTE

Lymphocytes are the second most common cell type in the peripheral blood of most of the domestic species and are the most common cell type in ruminants. In most of the common laboratory animal species, the percentage of the lymphocytes is greater than that of the neutrophils. Typically, these cells are round, slightly smaller than neutrophils, and have round to oval and sometimes slightly indented nuclei. The chromatin pattern consists of smooth glassy areas intermixed with areas that are more clumped or smudged. A small amount of light blue cytoplasm is present. A few of the lymphocytes may have multiple, small, pinkish-purple granules in the cytoplasm. These are commonly seen in rats. In guinea pigs, lymphocytes with a large eosinophilic cytoplasmic inclusion (Kurloff body) may be present in low numbers. These cells are called Kurloff cells and are thought to have natural killer cell function.

In addition to small lymphocytes, many animals may have some medium to large lymphocytes. This is especially true for ruminants. Often, these cells have more cytoplasm than small lymphocytes. In addition, the chromatin of ruminant nuclei is often much more accentuated with sometimes marked areas of condensation. This may lead to the false conclusion that nucleoli are present in these cells.

MONOCYTE

Monocytes are absent or present in low numbers in the peripheral blood and look very similar in all the common domestic species and laboratory animal species. These cells are typically 15–20 μm in diameter, and the nuclei can be different shapes, such as oval or oval with a single indentation (kidney bean–shaped), or have multiple indentations and lobulations. The nuclear chromatin is finely granular to lacy in appearance, with only a few areas of condensation. The moderate amount of cytoplasm is typically blue-gray and may have multiple, variably sized discrete vacuoles.

EOSINOPHIL

Eosinophils are absent or present in very low numbers in normal animals. These cells are typically similar in size than neutrophils but are often slightly larger. The nuclei are very similar to those of neutrophils in that they are segmented, but the segments are often not as well defined. The cytoplasm stains faint blue and has multiple reddish to reddish-orange granules. The numbers and shapes of the granules are quite different for most of the common domestic species. Dog eosinophilic granules are round and quite variable in size and number. There are often multiple, variably sized vacuoles in the cytoplasm as well. Cat eosinophilic granules are rod shaped and typically fill the cytoplasm. Horse eosinophils have very large round, oval, or oblong granules that fill the cytoplasm and often obscure the nucleus. Ruminant eosinophils have small round, fairly uniform granules that typically fill the cytoplasm. Llama eosinophils have small round, oval, or oblong granules. The low number of granules typically does not fill the cytoplasm. In the common laboratory animal species, the number of granules is variable. Ferret eosinophils look similar to dog eosinophils. Guinea pig and rabbit eosinophils have large round granules that often fill the cytoplasm. In nonhuman primates (cynomolgus monkey), the granules are rounded and larger than the granules in the neutrophil, and they fill the cytoplasm. In the rat and mouse, abundant round granules are present in the cytoplasm. Rat and mouse eosinophils are often less segmented, and ring shaped nuclei may be present.

BASOPHIL

Basophils are rarely seen in the peripheral blood of all the common domestic species. They are most commonly seen in horses. Basophils are similar in size or slightly larger than neutrophils, and the cytoplasm is light purple. The nucleus is segmented but often not to the degree of the mature neutrophil. Low numbers of small, round, purple cytoplasmic granules may sometimes be present in dog basophils. The presence or absence of granules may be dependent on the type of stain used. Cat basophils contain indistinct small, round, lavender granules. Both cow and horse basophils have several small, well-stained purple granules in the cytoplasm. Llama basophils look very similar to cow or horse basophils. Overall, the basophils of the common laboratory animal species look similar to those of the common domestic animal species. In the rabbit, these cells are more common than in most other species and are regularly seen in peripheral blood. The cells have abundant purple cytoplasmic granules. In rodents, mast cells can also be seen in low numbers in blood smears and probably represent contamination with tissue mast cells during certain types of collection procedures. These cells are larger than basophils and have round nuclei and abundant purple cytoplasmic granules that often obscure the nucleus.

Figures 5.1–5.66 show the normal white blood cells of the common domestic (canine, feline, equine, bovine, and llama) and laboratory animal (nonhuman primate [cynomolgus monkey], rabbit [New Zealand White], guinea pig, ferret, rat [Sprague Dawley], and mouse [CD1]) species.

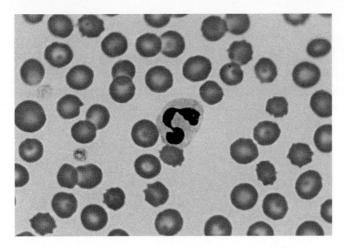

Figure 5.1 Segmented neutrophil. The cell with the segmented nucleus and pink cytoplasm is a mature neutrophil. Canine blood smear; 100× objective.

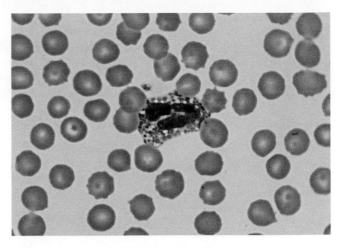

Figure 5.4 Eosinophil. The cell with a poorly segmented nucleus and multiple, round reddish granules in the cytoplasm is an eosinophil. Canine blood smear; 100× objective.

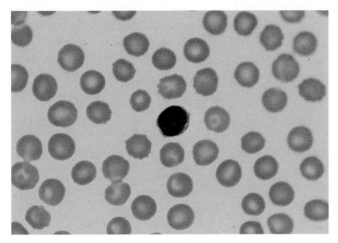

Figure 5.2 Small lymphocyte. The small cell with a round, centrally located nucleus and a rim of light blue cytoplasm is a small lymphocyte. Canine blood smear; 100× objective.

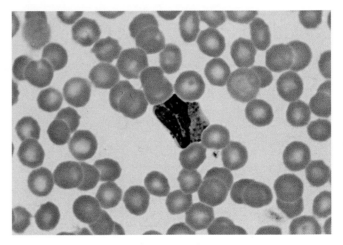

Figure 5.5 Basophil. The cell with the poorly segmented nucleus and light purple cytoplasm with low numbers of small, discrete purple granules is a basophil. Canine blood smear; 100× objective.

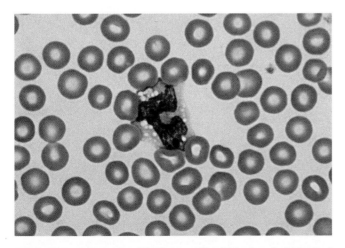

Figure 5.3 Monocyte. The large cell with a deeply indented nucleus; blue-gray cytoplasm; and multiple, discrete cytoplasmic vacuoles is a monocyte. Note that the nucleus is not as prominently segmented as the mature neutrophil. Canine blood smear; 100× objective.

Figure 5.6 Basophil. The cell with the poorly segmented nucleus and light purple cytoplasm is a basophil. Without distinct granules, these cells can be difficult to distinguish from toxic neutrophils or monocytes. Canine blood smear; 100× objective.

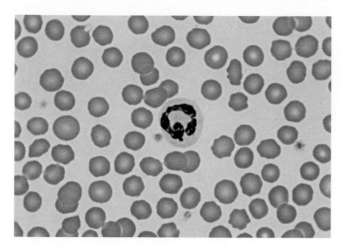

Figure 5.7 Segmented neutrophil. The cell with a segmented nucleus and light pink cytoplasm is a mature neutrophil. Feline blood smear; 100× objective.

Figure 5.10 Eosinophil. The cell with a segmented nucleus and multiple, reddish rod-shaped granules in the cytoplasm is an eosinophil. Feline blood smear; 100× objective.

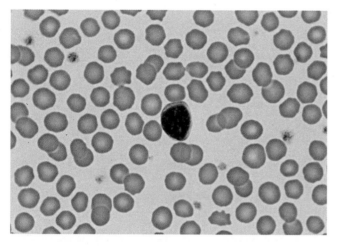

Figure 5.8 Small lymphocyte. The small cell with a round to oval, centrally located nucleus and a rim of light blue cytoplasm is a small lymphocyte. Feline blood smear; 100× objective.

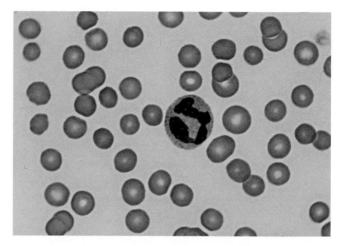

Figure 5.11 Basophil. The cell with a segmented nucleus and poorly defined, round, light purple granules in the cytoplasm is a basophil. Feline blood smear; 100× objective.

Figure 5.9 Monocyte. The large cell with a deeply indented nucleus, blue-gray cytoplasm, and multiple, discrete cytoplasmic vacuoles is a monocyte. Feline blood smear; 100× objective.

Figure 5.12 Segmented neutrophil and basophil. The cell to the lower left is a segmented neutrophil, and the cell to the upper right is a basophil. Note the slightly larger size of the basophil as well as the poorly defined, round, light purple cytoplasmic granules. Feline blood smear; 100× objective.

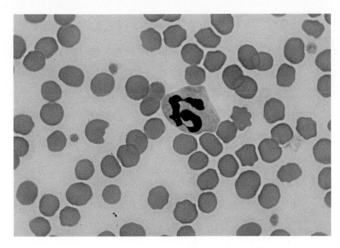

Figure 5.13 Segmented neutrophil. The cell with a segmented nucleus and light blue to pink cytoplasm is a mature neutrophil. Equine blood smear; 100× objective.

Figure 5.16 Eosinophil. The cell with the bilobed nucleus and very large, round to oval reddish granules in the cytoplasm is an eosinophil. Note that the granules are obscuring part of the nucleus. Equine blood smear; 100× objective.

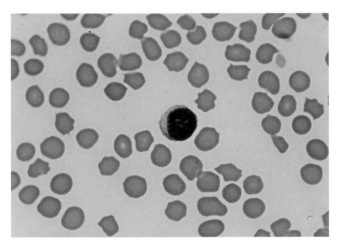

Figure 5.14 Small lymphocyte. The small cell with a round nucleus and a rim of light blue cytoplasm is a small lymphocyte. Equine blood smear; 100× objective.

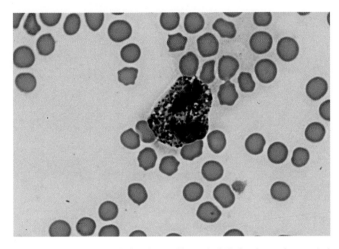

Figure 5.17 Basophil. The cell with bilobed nucleus and numerous small, purple cytoplasmic granules is a basophil. Note that the granules are obscuring part of the nucleus. Equine blood smear; 100× objective.

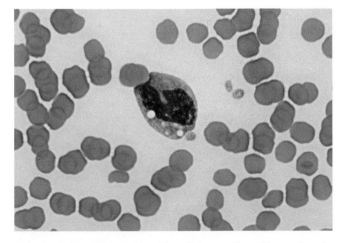

Figure 5.15 Monocyte. The large cell with a deeply indented nucleus; blue-gray cytoplasm; and multiple, discrete cytoplasmic vacuoles is a monocyte. Equine blood smear; 100× objective.

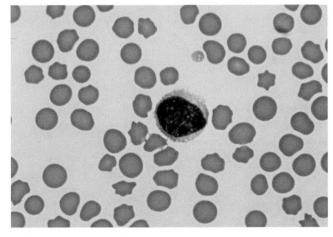

Figure 5.18 Large lymphocyte. The large round cell with an oval nucleus and a rim of light blue cytoplasm is a large lymphocyte. Equine blood smear; 100× objective.

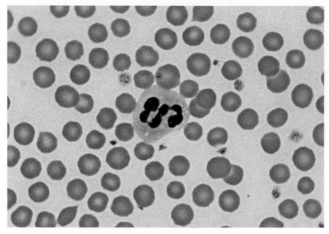

Figure 5.19 Segmented neutrophil. The cell with a segmented nucleus and light pink cytoplasm is a mature neutrophil. Bovine blood smear; 100× objective.

Figure 5.22 Eosinophil. The cell with the elongated nucleus and abundant, small, round reddish granules in the cytoplasm is an eosinophil. Bovine blood smear; 100× objective.

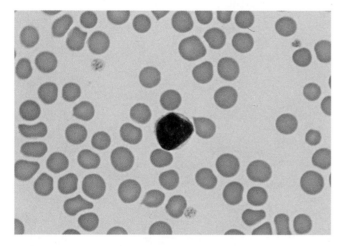

Figure 5.20 Small lymphocyte. The cell with the round to oval nucleus and a rim of light blue cytoplasm is a small lymphocyte. Bovine blood smear; 100× objective.

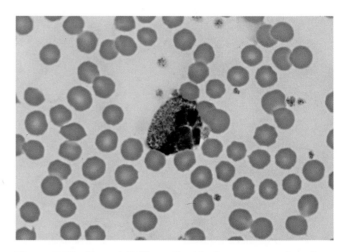

Figure 5.23 Basophil. The cell with the segmented nucleus and numerous, small purple granules in the cytoplasm is a basophil. Bovine blood smear; 100× objective.

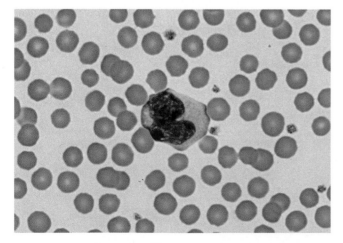

Figure 5.21 Monocyte. The large cell with the deeply indented nucleus and blue-gray cytoplasm is a monocyte. Note the lack of vacuoles; not all monocytes contain vacuoles. Bovine blood smear; 100× objective.

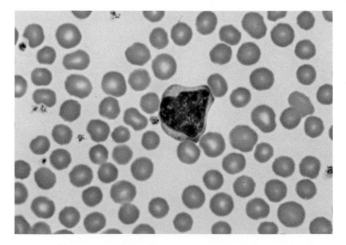

Figure 5.24 Large lymphocyte. The cell with a round to slightly indented nucleus with small amounts of light blue cytoplasm is a large lymphocyte. Note the accentuated nuclear chromatin pattern that is often seen in normal bovine lymphocytes. Bovine blood smear; 100× objective.

Figure 5.25 Neutrophils. The two cells with segmented nuclei and light blue to pink granular cytoplasm are segmented neutrophils. Llama blood smear; 100× objective.

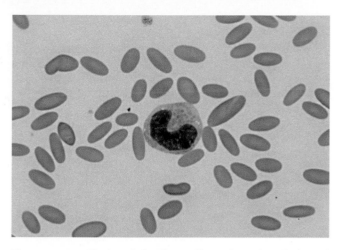

Figure 5.28 Eosinophil. The cell with a band-shaped nucleus and low numbers of poorly defined, small, round to oblong, reddish granules in the cytoplasm is an eosinophil. Often llama eosinophils have low numbers of cytoplasmic granules. Llama blood smear; 100× objective.

Figure 5.26 Small lymphocyte. The cell with the round nucleus and small amount of light blue cytoplasm is a small lymphocyte. Llama blood smear; 100× objective.

Figure 5.29 Basophil. The cell with the poorly segmented nucleus and multiple, small purple cytoplasmic granules is a basophil. The granules partially obscure the nucleus. Llama blood smear; 100× objective.

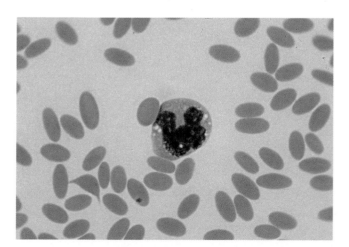

Figure 5.27 Monocyte. The large cell with a deeply indented nucleus, blue-gray cytoplasm, and multiple, discrete cytoplasmic vacuoles is a monocyte. Llama blood smear; 100× objective.

Figure 5.30 Eosinophil. The cell with a bilobed nucleus and multiple, round, reddish granules is a well-granulated eosinophil. Llama blood smear; 100× objective.

Figure 5.31 Segmented neutrophil. The cell with the segmented nucleus, light blue cytoplasm, and pink granules is a mature neutrophil. Rat blood smear; 100× objective.

Figure 5.34 Eosinophil and lymphocyte. The cell with the ring-shaped nucleus and multiple, round, reddish granules in the cytoplasm is an eosinophil. The small round cell to the left of the eosinophil is a lymphocyte. Rat blood smear; 100× objective.

Figure 5.32 Small lymphocyte. The small cell with a round nucleus and a rim of blue cytoplasm is a small lymphocyte. Rat blood smear; 100× objective.

Figure 5.35 Basophil. The cell with the poorly segmented nucleus and light purple cytoplasm with low numbers of small, discrete, purple granules is a basophil. Rat blood smear; 100× objective.

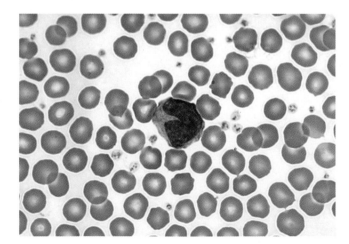

Figure 5.33 Monocyte. The large cell with a deeply indented nucleus and blue-gray cytoplasm is a monocyte. Rat blood smear; 100× objective.

Figure 5.36 Lymphocyte. The cell with the round to oblong nucleus and blue cytoplasm with prominent eosinophilic granules is a lymphocyte. It is common to see low numbers of granulated lymphocytes in rats. Rat blood smear; 100× objective.

Figure 5.37   Segmented neutrophil. The cell with the segmented nucleus, light blue cytoplasm, and indistinct pink granules is a mature neutrophil. Mouse blood smear; 100× objective.

Figure 5.40   Eosinophil. The cell with a poorly segmented nucleus and multiple, round reddish granules in the cytoplasm is an eosinophil. Mouse blood smear; 100× objective.

Figure 5.38   Small and large lymphocyte. The small cell in the right lower quadrant with a round nucleus and a rim of blue cytoplasm is a small lymphocyte. The large cell in the upper left quadrant with a round nucleus with a small amount of light blue cytoplasm is a large lymphocyte. Mouse blood smear; 100× objective.

Figure 5.41   Eosinophil. The cell with a ring-shaped nucleus and multiple, round, reddish granules in the cytoplasm is an eosinophil. Note that "ring form" eosinophils are common in mouse blood smears. Mouse blood smear; 100× objective.

Figure 5.39   Monocyte. The large cell in the upper right quadrant with a slightly indented nucleus, blue cytoplasm, and few vacuoles is a monocyte. The round cell in the lower left quadrant is a small lymphocyte. Mouse blood smear; 100× objective.

Figure 5.42   The cell with the round to oval nucleus and blue cytoplasm with eosinophilic granules is a granulated lymphocyte. Multiple platelets, often found on top of red blood cells, are also present. Inset lower right is a greater magnification. Mouse blood smear; 100× objective.

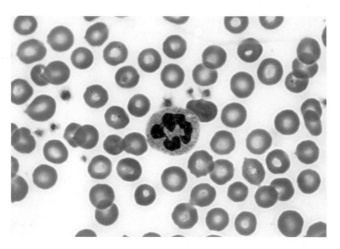

Figure 5.43 Segmented neutrophil. The cell with the segmented nucleus, light blue cytoplasm, and numerous small distinct pink granules is a mature neutrophil. Note that monkey neutrophils often have more nuclear segments than other species. Nonhuman primate (cynomolgus monkey) blood smear; 100× objective.

Figure 5.44 Small lymphocyte. The small cell with a round to oval nucleus and a rim of blue cytoplasm is a small lymphocyte. Nonhuman primate (cynomolgus monkey) blood smear; 100× objective.

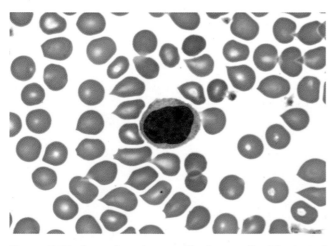

Figure 5.45 Large lymphocyte. The large cell with an oval to oblong nucleus and a rim of light blue cytoplasm is a large lymphocyte. Nonhuman primate (cynomolgus monkey) blood smear; 100× objective.

Figure 5.46 Monocyte. The large cell with an indented nucleus, blue cytoplasm, and few vacuoles is a monocyte. Nonhuman primate (cynomolgus monkey) blood smear; 100× objective.

Figure 5.47 Eosinophil. The cell with a poorly segmented nucleus and multiple, round, reddish granules in the cytoplasm is an eosinophil. Note that the granules obscure part of the nucleus, which makes it difficult to visualize its continuity. Nonhuman primate (cynomolgus monkey) blood smear; 100× objective.

Figure 5.48 Basophil and lymphocyte. The segmented cell (center) with light purple cytoplasm and purple cytoplasmic granules is a basophil. Note that the cell with a round nucleus to the right of the basophil is a small lymphocyte. Nonhuman primate (cynomolgus monkey) blood smear; 100× objective.

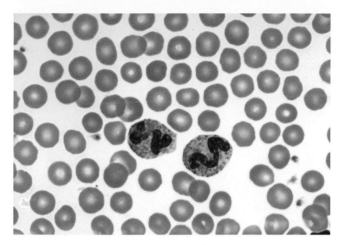

Figure 5.49 Heterophils. The cells with the segmented nuclei and distinct small, reddish granules are heterophils. Rabbit blood smear; 100× objective.

Figure 5.52 Eosinophil. The cell with a poorly segmented nucleus and multiple, large, round, reddish granules in the cytoplasm is an eosinophil. Rabbit blood smear; 100× objective.

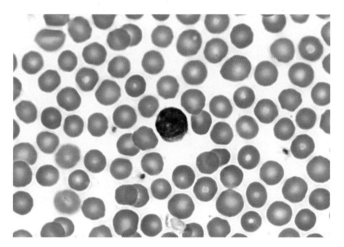

Figure 5.50 Small lymphocyte. The small cell with a round nucleus and a rim of blue cytoplasm is a small lymphocyte. Rabbit blood smear; 100× objective.

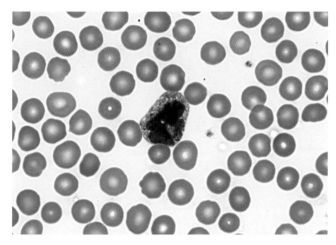

Figure 5.53 Basophil. The cell with the poorly segmented nucleus, purple foamy cytoplasm, and few distinct purple granules is a basophil. Rabbit blood smear; 100× objective.

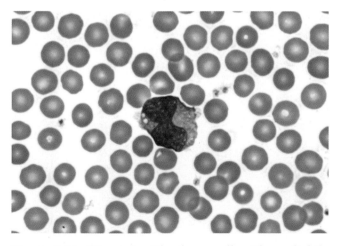

Figure 5.51 Monocyte. The large cell with a slightly indented nucleus, blue cytoplasm, and few vacuoles is a monocyte. Rabbit blood smear; 100× objective.

Figure 5.54 Basophil, heterophil, and eosinophil. The cell with the poorly segmented nucleus and light purple cytoplasm with low numbers of small, discrete, purple granules in the upper left is a basophil. The cell in the lower right with the segmented nucleus and distinct, small, reddish granules is a heterophil. The cell with multiple, large, round granules in the inset (upper right) is an eosinophil. Rabbit blood smear; 100× objective.

Figure 5.55 Segmented neutrophil. The cell with the segmented nucleus and distinct small reddish granules is a neutrophil. Guinea pig blood smear; 100× objective.

Figure 5.58 Eosinophil. The cell with a poorly segmented nucleus and multiple, large, round, reddish granules in the cytoplasm is an eosinophil. Note that the granules obscure part of the nucleus, which makes it difficult to visualize the continuity of the nucleus. Guinea pig blood smear; 100× objective.

Figure 5.56 Small lymphocyte. The small cell with a round nucleus and a rim of blue cytoplasm is a small lymphocyte. Guinea pig blood smear; 100× objective.

Figure 5.59 Basophil. The cell with abundant purple granules that fill the cytoplasm and obscure the nucleus is a basophil. Guinea pig blood smear; 100× objective.

Figure 5.57 Monocyte. The large cell with a slightly indented nucleus, blue cytoplasm, and few vacuoles is a monocyte. Guinea pig blood smear; 100× objective.

Figure 5.60 Lymphocyte with Kurloff body and neutrophil. The cell to the left with a partially indented nucleus and a large, round, pink cytoplasmic inclusion is a lymphocyte with a Kurloff body. A low number of Kurloff bodies can be found in normal guinea pigs. The cell to the right is a neutrophil. Guinea pig blood smear; 100× objective.

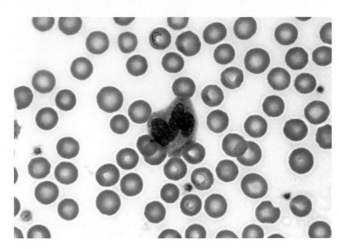

Figure 5.61 Segmented neutrophil. The cell with the segmented nucleus and light blue cytoplasm is a neutrophil. Ferret blood smear; 100× objective.

Figure 5.64 Eosinophil. The cell with a poorly segmented nucleus and multiple, small, round, reddish granules in the cytoplasm is an eosinophil. Ferret blood smear; 100× objective.

Figure 5.62 Small lymphocyte. The small cell with a round nucleus and a rim of blue cytoplasm is a small lymphocyte. Ferret blood smear; 100× objective.

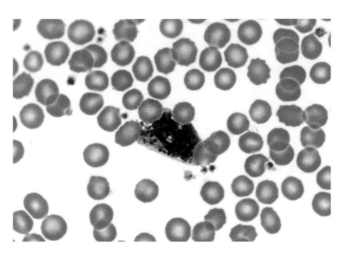

Figure 5.65 Basophil. The cell with the poorly segmented nucleus with moderate numbers of distinct purple granules in the cytoplasm is a basophil. Ferret blood smear; 100× objective.

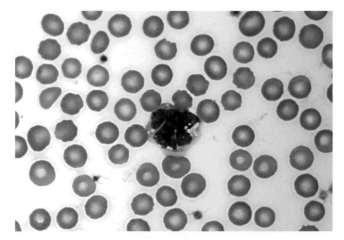

Figure 5.63 Monocyte. The large cell with multiple nuclear indentations, blue cytoplasm, and moderate numbers of vacuoles is a monocyte. Ferret blood smear; 100× objective.

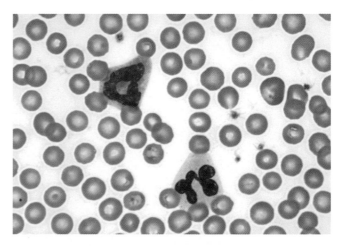

Figure 5.66 Eosinophil and neutrophil. The cell in the upper left is an eosinophil. The cell in the lower right is a neutrophil. Ferret blood smear; 100× objective.

CHAPTER SIX

VARIATIONS IN WHITE BLOOD CELL MORPHOLOGY

GRANULOCYTES

A common change that may be seen in animals with inflammation is the presence of increased numbers of immature neutrophilic granulocytes in the circulation. This is known as a left shift. Commonly, a left shift includes increased numbers of band neutrophils (Fig. 6.1), but it also may include metamyelocytes, myelocytes, and very rarely, promyelocytes and myeloblasts. The band neutrophils, as previously described, have hyposegmented nuclei. Typically, the chromatin of the band neutrophil is less condensed than that of the mature segmented neutrophil. In contrast, in Pelger-Huët anomaly, which has been reported in dogs, cats, rabbits, and horses, there is a defect that causes hyposegmentation of the granulocytes (Fig. 6.2) and results in the appearance of a false left shift. This condition is extremely rare but may be distinguished from a true left shift by the characteristics of the nuclear chromatin. In Pelger-Huët anomaly, although the cells are hyposegmented, the chromatin is very condensed, as in a normally segmented neutrophil. Transient pseudo–Pelger-Huët anomaly has also been reported in some disease states.

In all common domestic and laboratory animal species, during inflammation, neutrophilic granulocytes may appear in the blood with a group of morphological changes known as toxicity or toxic changes. These features are often present when there is a left shift. The three main features of toxicity that are seen include increased basophilia and foaminess and the presence of Döhle bodies in the cytoplasm. The basophilia of the cytoplasm is a result of an increased amount of ribosomal RNA (Figs. 6.3–6.5). The foaminess of the cytoplasm is thought to be caused by prominent lysosomes or dilated cytoplasmic organelles (Figs. 6.6 and 6.7). The Döhle bodies are irregularly shaped, small, blue-gray particles in the cytoplasm (Figs. 6.8 and 6.9). They are lamellar aggregates of rough endoplasmic reticulum. Döhle bodies in cats and horses are common during inflammation and, thus, are not considered as severe a sign of toxicity compared with in the other species. Depending on the degree and cause of the inflammation, there may be one or more features of toxicity present. One cause of severe toxicity is endotoxemia.

In addition to the three features mentioned above, another morphologic change that can be seen in toxic neutrophils is toxic granulation, which is the presence

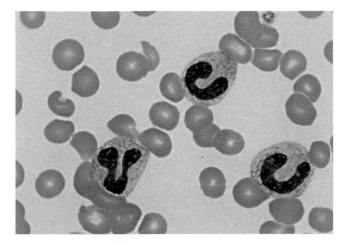

Figure 6.1 Band neutrophils. The two nucleated cells (right) are band neutrophils, and the cell in the lower left is a poorly segmented but more mature neutrophil. All of these cells are toxic, based on the increased bluish color and foaminess of the cytoplasm. Canine blood smear; 100× objective.

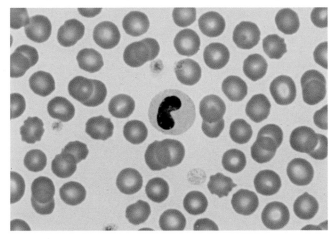

Figure 6.2 Pelger-Huët anomaly. The hyposegmented neutrophil with a very condensed chromatin pattern is typical of the Pelger-Huët anomaly. Canine blood smear; 100× objective.

of multiple, small, purple granules in the cytoplasm of the cell. These granules are probably prominent primary granules. This is not a common finding in the common domestic species but may rarely be seen in horses. Toxic granulation must be distinguished from inclusions in the neutrophils that may be seen in normal Birman cats, normal common laboratory animal species, and animals with lysosomal storage diseases.

Another rare morphological change that may be seen in animals with inflammation is the presence of giant neutrophils. These cells are produced and

released more rapidly from the bone marrow, and therefore, the normal maturation has not occurred—thus the larger size. Giant neutrophils may also be a sign of myelodysplasia, which is described in Chapter 9.

Other miscellaneous changes that may be seen in the granulocytes are neutrophilic hypersegmentation, variably sized eosinophilic granules, and eosinophilic degranulation. Hypersegmentation may be seen in all species and is defined in most species as neutrophils with more than five segments or lobules (Fig. 6.10). However, normal nonhuman primates (cynomolgus

Figure 6.3   Normal segmented neutrophil. Note the light pink cytoplasm compared with the blue cytoplasm in the toxic neutrophils in Figures 6.4 and 6.5. Feline blood smear; 100× objective.

Figure 6.5   Moderate to marked cytoplasmic basophilia. The poorly segmented neutrophil in the center of the field has moderate to marked toxicity, indicated by the presence of dark blue cytoplasm, foaminess of the cytoplasm, and Döhle bodies. Feline blood smear; 100× objective.

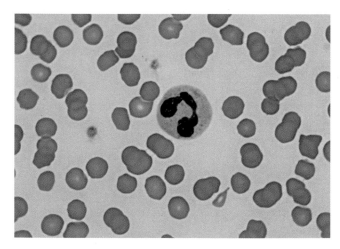

Figure 6.4   Mild to moderate cytoplasmic basophilia. The segmented neutrophil in the center of the field has mild to moderate toxicity, indicated by the presence of blue cytoplasm and Döhle bodies. Feline blood smear; 100× objective.

Figure 6.6   Mild cytoplasmic foaminess. There is mild foaminess of the cytoplasm of the poorly segmented neutrophil in the center of the field. Slight to moderate blue cytoplasm and Döhle bodies are also present, which further indicate moderate toxicity. Canine blood smear; 100× objective.

monkey) can commonly have up to eight segments. Hypersegmentation is typically a result of the retention of the cell in the circulation system much longer than normal, but it also can be seen when blood smears are not made soon enough after the blood has been collected. Hypersegmentation of the neutrophils also can occur in poodles with erythrocytic macrocytosis and giant schnauzers with B12 deficiency.

Marked variation in the size of the eosinophilic granules mainly occurs in dogs (Fig. 6.11). Some cells may be present with only a few larger granules and variable numbers of vacuoles.

Eosinophils with abundant vacuoles and no granules may be seen in dogs, with greyhounds being the most common breed in which these cells are easily identified. These cells are often incorrectly interpreted as toxic neutrophils. The distinguishing features of these eosinophils are that these cells are larger than neutrophils and often have multiple, discrete, variably sized vacuoles in the cytoplasm (Fig. 6.12).

Figure 6.7 Marked cytoplasmic foaminess. The cell to the right is a band neutrophil. The cell in the center is a metamyelocyte. The cell to the left is a lymphocyte. Both the band neutrophil and metamyelocyte show signs of marked toxicity resulting from the marked cytoplasmic foaminess and blue cytoplasm. Bovine blood smear; 100× objective.

Figure 6.9 Döhle bodies. The neutrophil has at least three Döhle bodies (irregular aggregates of blue material) at the two, eight, and ten o'clock positions in the cytoplasm. The pink cytoplasmic granules are normally present in nonhuman primate neutrophils. Nonhuman primate (cynomolgus monkey) blood smear; 100× objective.

Figure 6.8 Döhle body. The irregular aggregate of blue material at the twelve o'clock position in the cytoplasm of the segmented neutrophil (center) is a Döhle body. Moderate basophilia and mild cytoplasmic foaminess are also present. Feline blood smear; 100× objective.

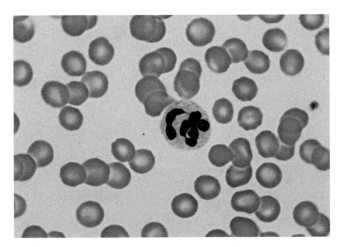

Figure 6.10 Hypersegmented neutrophil. The nucleus of the neutrophil in the center of the field has seven lobules. A cell with five or more nuclear lobules is considered hypersegmented. Canine blood smear; 100× objective.

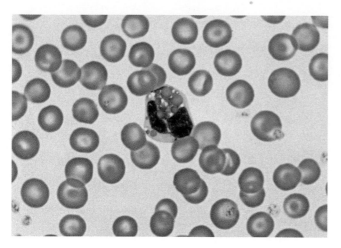

Figure 6.11 Eosinophil with large, variably sized granules. The nucleated cell (center) is an eosinophil with large, variably sized, reddish granules. Canine blood smear; 100× objective.

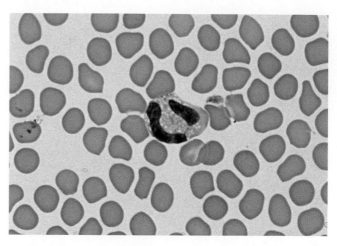

Figure 6.12 Degranulated eosinophil. The cell in the center of the field with a bilobed nucleus joined by a thin filament and multiple, variably sized, poorly defined vacuoles is a degranulated greyhound eosinophil. Canine blood smear; 100× objective.

AGRANULOCYTES

The major different morphological changes that occur in the agranulocytes are variations in the morphology of lymphocytes. Reactive lymphocytes, also known as immunocytes, are typically lymphocytes with dark blue cytoplasm and possibly increased amounts of cytoplasm (Figs. 6.13–6.15). These cells may also have a prominent perinuclear clear zone. Low numbers of reactive lymphocytes can be found in normal animals but typically are found in increased numbers in animals that are antigenically stimulated.

Plasma cells or plasmacytoid reactive lymphocytes are rarely seen in the peripheral blood (Fig. 6.16). These cells have much more cytoplasm than normal, or reactive, lymphocytes. The cytoplasm is deep blue to blue-green. Often there is a prominent perinuclear clear zone. The nucleus is round with marked condensation of the chromatin in some areas and clear in other areas. Rarely, these cells may have multiple discrete inclusions in the cytoplasm, known as Russell bodies.

Atypical lymphocyte is a term that is used differently by different people. We describe atypical lymphocytes as those cells with a morphology similar to that of reactive lymphocytes, but in addition to dark blue cytoplasm, and possibly increased amounts of cytoplasm, there are nuclear abnormalities. In contrast to normal lymphocytes, in which the nucleus is round to slightly indented, the nucleus of atypical lymphocytes has deep clefts or multiple indentations or infoldings (Fig. 6.17). The presence of a rare atypical lymphocyte may be associated with just antigenic stimulation. However, the presence of high numbers of these cells may indicate that the animal has a lymphoproliferative disorder (see Chapter 9).

Lymphoblasts are lymphocytes with nuclei that contain one or more nucleoli (Fig. 6.18). These cells typically are much larger than small lymphocytes, although small lymphoblasts may be seen. Not only does the nucleus of a lymphoblast contain a prominent nucleolus but the chromatin also is more open and finely stippled compared with that of the normal small lymphocyte. If lymphoblasts are easy to find in the peripheral blood, the animal most likely has a lymphoproliferative disorder. Because of the marked accentuation of the chromatin of the normal bovine large lymphocyte, these cells are often misinterpreted as lymphoblasts.

Normal monocytic morphology has been previously described. The major variation in monocytic morphology is that some monocytes lack prominent vacuoles (Figs. 6.19 and 6.20). This can occur in any species. When these cells lack vacuoles, they may be confused with band neutrophils or atypical lymphocytes. Usually, if there is any question in interpretation, more-typical monocytes with vacuoles can be found on the blood smear, and these cells can be useful in confirming that the cells without vacuoles are truly monocytes. In addition, the chromatin of the monocyte is more granular to lacy, with some areas of condensation, compared with the more condensed chromatin of the band neutrophil.

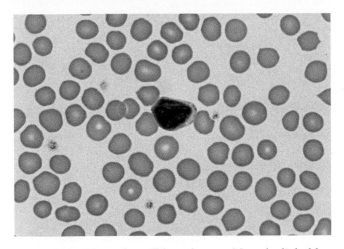

Figure 6.13 Normal small lymphocyte. Note the light blue cytoplasm compared with the dark blue cytoplasm of the reactive lymphocytes in Figures 6.14 and 6.15. Feline blood smear; 100× objective.

Figure 6.16 Plasmacytoid reactive lymphocyte. The lymphocyte has abundant dark blue cytoplasm with eccentrically placed round nucleus, perinuclear clear zone, and few vacuoles. Nonhuman primate (cynomolgus monkey) blood smear; 100× objective.

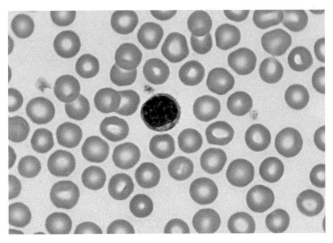

Figure 6.14 Reactive lymphocyte. The dark blue cytoplasm and poorly defined, perinuclear clear zone are typical of a reactive lymphocyte. Canine blood smear; 100× objective.

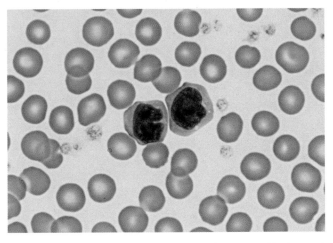

Figure 6.17 Atypical lymphocytes. The two cells (center) with deeply clefted nuclei and dark blue cytoplasm are atypical lymphocytes. Canine blood smear; 100× objective.

Figure 6.15 Reactive lymphocyte. This lymphocyte has increased amounts of dark blue cytoplasm, which is supportive of reactivity. Ferret blood smear; 100× objective.

Figure 6.18 Lymphoblasts. The three largest cells with round to oval nuclei, single or multiple nucleoli, and small amounts of blue cytoplasm are lymphoblasts. Canine blood smear; 100× objective.

Figure 6.19   Monocyte. The large cell (center) with a deeply indented nucleus and blue-gray cytoplasm with no cytoplasmic vacuoles is a monocyte. Note the pale, finely granular nuclear chromatin compared with the condensed chromatin of the toxic band neutrophil (top center). There is also a toxic segmented neutrophil present (lower left), as well as metarubricytes (top left and right corners). Canine blood smear; 100× objective.

Figure 6.20   Monocyte. The large cell (center) with a deeply indented nucleus and blue-gray cytoplasm is a monocyte. Note the multiple, discrete, clear, cytoplasmic vacuoles in the monocyte compared with the monocyte in Figure 6.19; these photomicrographs are from the same blood smear. A metarubricyte is present (lower right), and a red blood cell with basophilic stippling is present (upper left). Canine blood smear; 100× objective.

CHAPTER SEVEN

WHITE BLOOD CELL
INCLUSIONS AND PARASITES

Overall, the presence of inclusions or parasites in white blood cells is a much less common finding than that of inclusions or parasites in red blood cells. In addition, if inclusions or parasites are present, they are often present in extremely low numbers.

Azurophilic granules, which may be confused with viral inclusions or parasites, are present in some normal lymphocytes. These typically small, variably sized, and often multiple pink to purple granules can be found in lymphocytes of any species (Fig. 7.1). Rarely, these granules can be quite large, especially in ruminants and rats. In most normal animals, only a small percentage of lymphocytes are granulated. The llama and rat commonly have lymphocytes with granules. Large prominent single inclusions (Kurloff bodies) in lymphocytes are also present in guinea pigs and should not be confused with organisms (Fig. 5.60).

Organisms can be found in the white blood cells of dogs with ehrlichiosis. The *Ehrlichia* morulae can be a few to several microns in diameter. Each morula is relatively well formed and is made up of multiple, small, blue to purple coccoid structures known as elementary bodies. When morulae are present in monocytes or lymphocytes, they are often *Ehrlichia canis*, found mainly in tropical and subtropical areas.

Morulae that are present in neutrophils or eosinophils are typically *Ehrlichia ewingii* (Fig. 7.2) or *Anaplasma phagocytophilum* (Fig. 7.3). The morulae of *A. phagocytophilum* are generally less organized, and potentially, only very few blue to purple coccoid structures may be present.

Figure 7.2 Morula of *Ehrlichia ewingii*. The neutrophil in the center of the field has a single cytoplasmic morula. Canine buffy coat smear, courtesy of D. Boon; 100× objective.

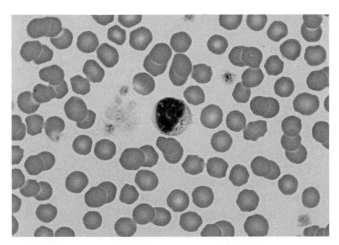

Figure 7.1 Azurophilic granules. The lymphocyte has several small, pink to purple cytoplasmic granules adjacent to the nucleus. Feline blood smear; 100× objective.

Figure 7.3 *Anaplasma phagocytophilum.* The neutrophil in the center of the field has multiple deep blue coccoid inclusions typical of *A. phagocytophilum.* Inset (upper left), greater magnification. Canine blood smear; 100× objective.

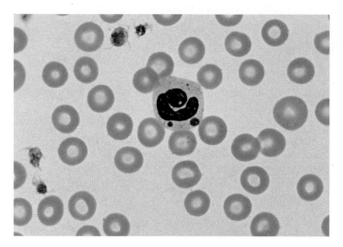

Figure 7.4 Canine distemper viral inclusions. The segmented neutrophil in the center of the field has prominent, round, light purple cytoplasmic inclusions characteristic of canine distemper virus. Canine blood smear; 100× objective.

Figure 7.5 *Hepatozoon canis.* The neutrophil in the center of the field has a single, large, oblong cytoplasmic structure with eccentrically placed, purple granular material. This is a gametocyte of *H. canis.* The inset in the upper right of the field is another neutrophil from the same blood film. This neutrophil has both a *H. canis* gametocyte as well as a well formed morula of *Ehrlichia canis.* Canine blood smear; 100× objective.

Distemper viral inclusions in dogs can potentially be found in all types of white blood cells. They are quite variable in size and stain pink to light purple. These round, oval to oblong, irregular structures have from a granular to often a smooth, glassy appearance (Fig. 7.4). Single or multiple inclusions may be present.

Hepatozoon canis is typically found in neutrophils or monocytes. Cases have been mainly reported in the U.S. Gulf Coast states, France, Italy, the Middle East, and Asia. *H. canis* gametocytes are large, oblong to oval organisms, typically measuring 5–10 μm and stain light blue (Fig. 7.5).

Histoplasma capsulatum can be found in neutrophils, monocytes, and eosinophils in the United States, and sporadically elsewhere. They are 2–4 μm in diameter and are round to oval structures (Fig. 7.6). They stain light blue and contain pink to purple, eccentrically placed granular nuclear material. Often there is a small halo around the organism. Single or multiple organisms may be present.

Mucopolysaccharidoses are a group of uncommon lysosomal storage diseases found in cats as well as dogs. Mucopolysaccharidoses types I, VI, and VII in cats and type VII in dogs have been reported to have pinpoint purple granules in the cytoplasm of neutrophils (Fig. 7.7). Cats with GM_2 gangliosidosis, another lysosomal storage disease, also have neutrophil granulation. Granulation may be seen in other white blood cell types in these disorders as well. Granulation of the lysosomal storage disease can look similar to toxic granulation but may be distinguished from it because

Figure 7.6 *Histoplasma capsulatum.* The monocyte/macrophage has three light blue oval organisms with purple, eccentrically placed granular material. These are *H. capsulatum* organisms. Canine blood smear, feathered edge; 100× objective.

there are typically no other signs of toxicity in the neutrophils. Biochemical testing is required to confirm the type of lysosomal storage disease. Similar granulation has been seen in neutrophils in some Birman cats. These cats do not have clinical signs that are typically associated with lysosomal storage diseases.

Certain types of lysosomal storage diseases in cats, including Nieman-Pick disease, gangliosidosis, mucopolysaccharidosis, and mannosidosis, result in vacu-

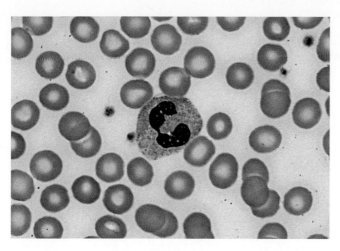

Figure 7.7 Mucopolysaccharidosis type VI. The neutrophil in the center of the field has multiple, small, light purple granules in the cytoplasm; this is typical of mucopolysaccharidosis type VI. Feline blood smear; 100× objective.

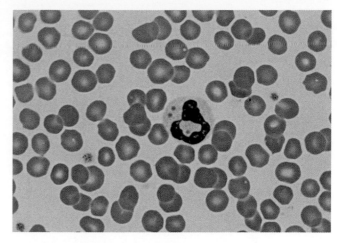

Figure 7.9 Chédiak-Higashi syndrome. The neutrophil in the center of the field has three small, round, pink cytoplasmic granules typical of Chédiak-Higashi syndrome. Feline blood smear, from 1987 American Society for Veterinary Clinical Pathology slide review, courtesy of M. Menard; 100× objective.

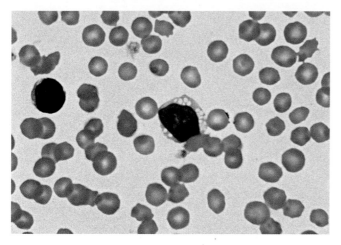

Figure 7.8 Gangliosidosis. The lymphocyte in the center of the field has multiple, variably sized, discrete cytoplasmic vacuoles typical of some lysosomal storage diseases, including gangliosidosis. The lymphocyte to the left is more normal appearing. Feline blood smear, from 1988 American Society for Veterinary Clinical Pathology slide review, courtesy of S. Dial; 100× objective.

olation of white blood cells. These multiple, small discrete vacuoles are most easily recognized in lymphocytes (Fig. 7.8). In some of these storage diseases, granules may also be found inside a portion of the vacuoles. Biochemical characterization of the enzyme deficiency is necessary to confirm and accurately classify the disorder. Fresh blood smears should be examined because vacuolation of normal white blood cells may also occur over time in vitro. Vacuolation of neutrophils has also been reported in cats after administration of high doses of chloramphenicol and phenylbutazone.

Another rare hereditary disorder of cats in which leukocyte inclusions may be present is Chédiak-Higashi syndrome (Fig. 7.9). The granules are typically round to oval, ranging in size from 2 μm in diameter to slightly larger. They stain light pink, and single or multiple granules may be present.

Inclusions and parasites in white blood cells of horses are uncommon. *Ehrlichia equi* (mainly found in the United States), now known as *Anaplasma phagocytophilum*, looks similar to *Ehrlichia canis* and typically can be found in neutrophils, but rarely in eosinophils.

Inclusions and parasites in white blood cells of cattle are also uncommon. *A. phagocytophilum* is reported in Northern and Western Europe. The rare hereditary disorder, Chédiak-Higashi syndrome, has been reported in cattle and looks similar to the inclusions described for cats.

Vacuolation of cow as well as sheep lymphocytes has been reported in the lysosomal storage disease known as acquired alpha mannosidosis. The decrease in the enzyme activity of alpha mannosidase is caused by the ingestion of swainsonine, which is found in the locoweed plant. Measurement of swainsonine in the blood can be done to confirm this disease.

As a result of the controlled environment in which laboratory animals are usually kept, a parasitic inclusion in the white blood cells does not occur frequently. Acquired lysosomal storage diseases in rats, and potentially other common laboratory animal species,

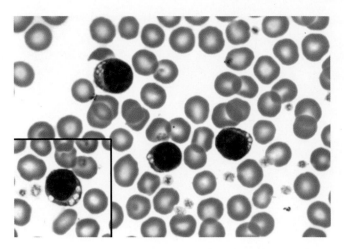

Figure 7.10   Phospholipidosis. The three lymphocytes have few to multiple, small, variably sized cytoplasmic vacuoles typical of phospholipidosis. Inset (lower left) demonstrates a lymphocyte with more prominent vacuoles. Rat blood smear; 100× objective.

Figure 7.12   Bacteria. The neutrophil in the center has multiple rod-shaped bacteria. Rat blood smear; 100× objective.

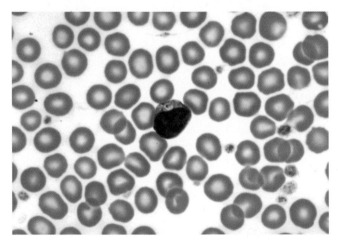

Figure 7.11   Phospholipidosis. The lymphocyte in the center of the field has a few variably sized cytoplasmic vacuoles containing granules. Granules may be found in some of the lymphocytes in rats with phospholipidosis. Rat blood smear; 100× objective.

Figure 7.13   Bacteria. The neutrophil in lower center of the field contains abundant coccoid bacteria. Four additional neutrophils are present. Nonhuman primate blood smear (cynomolgus monkey); 100× objective.

can be seen in animals treated with compounds that induce phospholipidosis. This results in lymphocytes with few to multiple variably sized cytoplasmic vacuoles (Fig. 7.10). Granules may sometimes be found inside a portion of the vacuoles (Fig. 7.11). Occasionally, bacteria may be found phagocytized in neutrophils (Figs. 7.12 and 7.13) in animals with severe bacterial infections.

CHAPTER EIGHT

PLATELETS

Platelets, also known as thrombocytes, morphologically look very similar in the common domestic and laboratory animal species, although in horses they generally do not stain as intensely (Figs. 8.1–8.7). Platelets are small, anucleated, discoid-shaped, light blue staining cells that may have multiple, fine, pink to purple granules in the cytoplasm. They are typi-

cally 2–4 µm in diameter. Rodent platelet counts are often much greater compared with the other species. Sometimes, if platelets are activated during the collection procedure, they may have multiple fine projections. If enough of the platelets are activated, they will coalesce and form large clumps (Fig. 8.6). It is sometimes difficult to make out the individual platelets in

Figure 8.1 Dog platelets. The small, round to oval, light blue anucleated cells with pink to purple cytoplasmic granules are platelets. Canine blood smear; 100× objective.

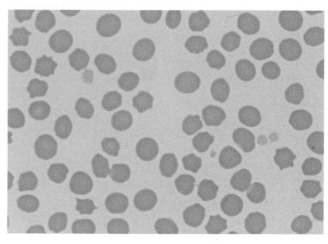

Figure 8.3 Horse platelets. The small, round to oval, very light blue anucleated cells with indistinct, pink cytoplasmic granules are platelets. These cells typically do not stain as intensely in horses as they do in other species. Equine blood smear; 100× objective.

Figure 8.2 Cat platelets. The small, round to oval, light blue anucleated cells with pink to purple cytoplasmic granules are platelets. Note the larger size of some of the platelets that are common in cats. Feline blood smear; 100× objective.

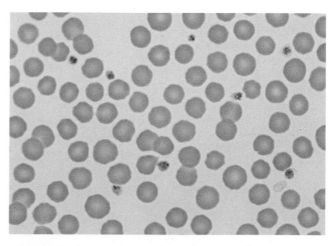

Figure 8.4 Cow platelets. The small, round to oval, light blue anucleated cells with pink to purple cytoplasmic granules are platelets. Bovine blood smear; 100× objective.

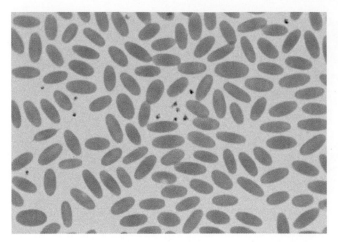

Figure 8.5 Llama platelets. The very small, round to oval, light blue anucleated cells with pink to purple cytoplasmic granules are platelets. Llama blood smear; 100× objective.

Figure 8.7 Macroplatelets. Two giant, or macro-, platelets are present (arrows). Canine blood smear; 100× objective.

Figure 8.6 Large platelet clump. A large irregular clump of platelets is present (center). Note the size of the platelet clump compared with the size of the neutrophil that is also present. Feline blood smear, feathered edge; 50× objective.

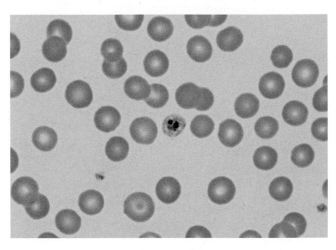

Figure 8.8 *Anaplasma platys*. The large platelet in the center of the field has two small, dark purple inclusions that are morulae of *A. platys*. Canine blood smear, from 1986 American Society for Veterinary Clinical Pathology slide review, courtesy of S. Gaunt; 100× objective.

these clumps. Often, because of their large size, platelet clumps can be found on the feathered edge of the slide.

With an increased demand for platelets, larger platelets may be released from the bone marrow. These larger platelets are known as macroplatelets, or giant platelets (Fig. 8.7). These platelets typically can be 5 μm or larger. Macroplatelets are commonly seen in feline peripheral blood samples, irrespective of disease state; in this species, this finding is not necessarily related to bone marrow response to a peripheral demand for platelets.

A rickettsial organism that has an affinity for platelets is *Anaplasma platys*, formerly known as *Ehrlichia platys*. Infection by this organism causes a disease that occurs in dogs mainly in the southern and southeastern portions of the United States and elsewhere in tropical and subtropical areas. The morphology of these organisms is similar to that of the *Anaplasma* species that infects white blood cells. The morulae are a few microns in diameter and are made up of multiple, small, blue to purple, coccoid-shaped structures known as elementary bodies (Fig. 8.8).

CHAPTER NINE

LYMPHOPROLIFERATIVE AND MYELOPROLIFERATIVE DISORDERS

GENERAL FEATURES

Animals with lymphoproliferative or myeloproliferative disorders have clonal proliferation of neoplastic cells of the lymphoid and myeloid lineage, respectively. When this neoplastic proliferation occurs in the bone marrow and these cells are released into the circulation, this is known as leukemia. The diagnosis of leukemia depends on several different factors, including history, clinical signs, and physical examination, as well as a detailed examination of the blood and bone marrow. Overall lymphoproliferative disorders are more common than myeloproliferative disorders, and with few exceptions (i.e., Fischer 344 rats), they both occur more frequently in common domestic species compared with common laboratory animal species.

Recently, the animal leukemia study group of the American Society for Veterinary Clinical Pathology proposed that an adaptation of the French/American/British classification scheme of leukemias of people be used in the classification of myeloid leukemias of dogs and cats. This system is based on recognizing the abnormal cells that are present, as well as systematically counting the different cell types present in the bone marrow. This classification scheme, although very useful, is beyond the scope of this atlas and is not used extensively here. Instead, the basic morphological approach is given for both lymphoid and myeloid leukemia. The discussion in this chapter focuses on those changes that are present in the peripheral blood of animals with leukemia, but again, this clearly is only one factor to consider in recognizing and classifying leukemias.

Finding an abnormality in the peripheral blood is often the first indication that leukemia may be present. With poorly differentiated leukemia, identification of a leukemic process is often easy; the difficulty lies in the proper classification. It is common in these cases to use the morphological assessment, cytochemical stains, molecular analysis, and immunophenotyping to properly identify the cell lineage/differentiation of the neoplastic cells. In contrast, in well-differentiated leukemia, the cell lineage is easy to recognize, but the challenge is to differentiate the leukemic process from inflammation.

LYMPHOPROLIFERATIVE DISORDERS

Lymphocytic Leukemia

Lymphocytic leukemia in the common domestic animal species occurs more frequently in dogs and cats compared with horses, cattle, and llamas. Lymphocytic leukemia can be divided into two major types: acute and chronic. Molecular analysis is becoming commonly used to differentiate T- and B-cell lymphocytic leukemia and is important in prognosis. This assessment cannot be made on morphology alone.

Acute Lymphocytic Leukemia Animals with acute lymphocytic leukemia, also known as acute lymphoblastic leukemia, often have high numbers of neoplastic cells in the circulation, but the morphology of these lymphocytes is not typical of those found in the circulation of a normal animal. In acute lymphocytic leukemia, the predominant cell type is a large, immature-appearing lymphocyte, typically a lymphoblast (Figs. 9.1 and 9.2).

Chronic Lymphocytic Leukemia In chronic lymphocytic leukemia, the predominant cell type is a cytomorphologically normal lymphocyte. These lymphocytes usually look similar to typical small- to medium-sized lymphocytes present in the circulation, but they are present in very high numbers (Figs. 9.3 and 9.4).

Lymphosarcoma

Neoplastic lymphocytes also may be found in the circulation during the leukemic phase of lymphosarcoma

Figure 9.1 Acute lymphocytic leukemia. Many large lymphocytes, often with prominent nucleoli, are present. Note the large size of these cells relative to the normal neutrophil in the left center of the field. Canine blood smear; 50× objective.

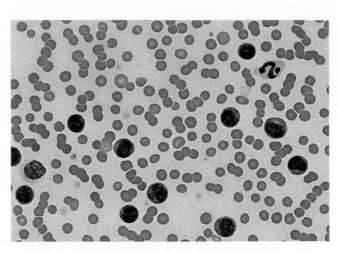

Figure 9.3 Chronic lymphocytic leukemia. Many small- to medium-sized lymphocytes are present in this field. One segmented neutrophil is in the upper right corner. Feline blood smear; 50× objective.

Figure 9.2 Acute lymphocytic leukemia. This is a greater magnification of the blood smear shown in Figure 9.1. Three large lymphocytes are present with prominent multiple nucleoli; these are lymphoblasts. A normal neutrophil is present in the upper-right corner. Canine blood smear; 100× objective.

Figure 9.4 Chronic lymphocytic leukemia. This is a greater magnification of the blood smear shown in Figure 9.3. Note the four small- to medium-sized lymphocytes that are normal to slightly reactive in morphology. Feline blood smear; 100× objective.

(Fig. 9.5). Lymphosarcoma is a lymphoproliferative disorder in which, typically, the neoplastic lymphocyte proliferation starts in primary sites other than the bone marrow, such as lymph nodes and tissues. In certain cases, the proliferation of the neoplastic cells will spread to the bone marrow, and subsequently to the blood, leading to the leukemic phase of lymphosarcoma. Because of the greater incidence of lymphosarcoma than acute lymphocytic leukemia, circulating lymphoblasts are more commonly seen with lymphosarcoma.

Large Granular Lymphocytic Leukemia

Another rare lymphoproliferative disorder that is unique as a result of the morphology of the lymphocytes is large granular lymphocytic leukemia (Figs. 9.6 and 9.7). As the name implies, these cells are large, with variably sized, purple cytoplasmic granules. This is a common leukemia seen in older Fischer 344 rats and is also referred to as mononuclear cell leukemia (Fig. 9.8).

Figure 9.5 Lymphoblasts. Seven large lymphocytes are present, often with prominent nucleoli; these are lymphoblasts. This animal is in the leukemic phase of lymphosarcoma. Bovine blood smear; 100× objective.

Figure 9.6 Large granular lymphocytic leukemia. Many large lymphocytes, often with prominent nucleoli, are present. Several of the cells also have large, round to irregularly shaped, purple cytoplasmic granules. Canine blood smear, from 1989 American Society for Veterinary Clinical Pathology slide review, courtesy of M. Wellman; 50× objective.

Figure 9.7 Large granular lymphocytic leukemia. This is a greater magnification of the blood smear shown in Figure 9.6. All the nucleated cells are large lymphocytes with often prominent nucleoli. Two of the cells have round to irregularly shaped, purple cytoplasmic granules. Canine blood smear, from 1989 American Society for Veterinary Clinical Pathology slide review, courtesy of M. Wellman; 100× objective.

Figure 9.8 Mononuclear cell leukemia (Large granular lymphocytic leukemia). Four large lymphocytes are present, with the lymphocyte located in the left center of the field containing purple cytoplasmic granules. Inset (lower left) is a lymphoblast. Note the nucleolus (basophilic ring structure) in the center of the nucleus. Rat blood smear (Fischer 344 rat); 100× objective.

Plasma Cell Myeloma

Finally, a lymphoproliferative disorder in which the neoplastic proliferation mainly occurs in the bone marrow is plasma cell myeloma. Plasma cells are seen in the circulation with this disorder. Plasma cells are not typically found in the circulation in animals with inflammatory disease, and thus, if they are present in high numbers, plasma cell myeloma should be considered.

MYELOPROLIFERATIVE DISORDERS

General Features

As with lymphoproliferative disorders, myeloproliferative disorders are more common in dogs and cats than in large animals. These disorders are most commonly recognized in cats and are often associated with feline leukemia virus infection. Myeloproliferative disorders involve cells of the granulocytic, monocytic, erythrocytic, and megakaryocytic lineages. Myeloproliferative disorders can be divided into three main categories: myelodysplastic syndrome, acute myeloid leukemia, and chronic myeloid leukemia. Myeloid leukemia can be a neoplastic proliferation of cells of single, as well as multiple, lineages.

Myelodysplastic Syndrome

Myelodysplastic syndrome is most often seen in cats. Myelodysplastic syndrome is also known as preleukemia, for animals with myelodysplastic syndrome may go on to develop myeloid leukemia. Although all animals with myelodysplastic syndrome will not progress to leukemia, it is still a life-threatening condition. As with leukemia, the diagnosis of myelodysplastic syndrome depends on multiple factors including history, clinical signs, physical examination, and a detailed examination of the blood and bone marrow; repeated examination of the blood, over time, is often necessary. Animals with myelodysplastic syndrome have abnormalities in the maturation of one or more myeloid lineage cell types. These maturation abnormalities are known as myelodysplasia. In addition, blast cells may be found in the circulation (Fig. 9.9). Cells with maturation abnormalities and blast

cells can also be found in the peripheral blood of animals with acute myeloid leukemia. The differentiation between these two processes is mainly a result of the number and type of abnormal cells present in the blood and bone marrow. Some myelodysplastic features found in the blood are described subsequently. Any given animal with myelodysplastic syndrome or myeloid leukemia may have one or more of these features.

Myelodysplasia of cells of the erythrocytic lineage is known as dyserythropoiesis. One feature of dyserythropoiesis is the formation of megaloblastic erythroid cells. These cells are recognized by their large size and asynchrony of maturation of the nucleus and cytoplasm. These cells often have mature-appearing, reddish-orange cytoplasm, which is typical of red blood cells with their full hemoglobin content, and a large, immature-appearing nucleus with uncondensed nuclear chromatin (Fig. 9.10). Megaloblastosis also can be seen with B12 and folate deficiency, but this rarely has been documented in the common domestic animals.

A second feature of dyserythropoiesis is macrocytosis, which is characterized by high numbers of macrocytes, large red blood cells, in circulation (Fig. 9.11). Macrocytosis is commonly seen in regenerative anemias in all animals, but in myelodysplasia, macrocytosis typically occurs concurrent with a nonregen-

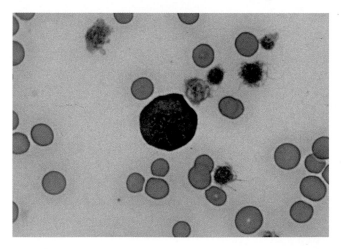

Figure 9.9 Blast cell. Low numbers of blast cells may be found in the circulation of animals with myelodysplastic syndrome. The nucleated cell (center) with the round eccentrically placed nucleus, prominent single nucleolus, and moderate amounts of blue cytoplasm is a blast cell of probable erythrocytic origin. Large platelets are present also. Feline blood smear; 100× objective.

Figure 9.10 Megaloblastic, nucleated red blood cell. The large cell (center) with slightly eccentric, relatively immature, ovoid nucleus with condensed chromatin and bluish-red cytoplasm is a megaloblastic red blood cell precursor. The giant size and asynchrony in maturation of the cytoplasm and nucleus are features of dyserythropoiesis. Large platelets are also present. Feline blood smear; 100× objective.

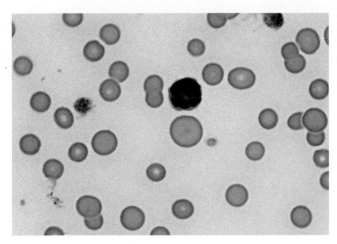

Figure 9.11   Macrocyte. The large, mature red blood cell in the center of the field directly below the lymphocyte is a macrocyte. Note the similarity of the size of this cell and the lymphocyte. If high numbers of macrocytes are present in an anemic animal with lack of polychromatophils, this is a feature of dyserythropoiesis. Feline blood smear; 100× objective.

Figure 9.13   Giant neutrophil. The segmented neutrophil in the upper left corner is larger than the adjacent segmented neutrophil and metamyelocyte in the lower portion of the field. This may be a feature of dysgranulopoiesis. Feline blood smear; 100× objective.

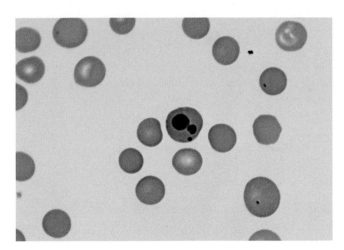

Figure 9.12   Abnormal nuclear shape. The metarubricyte in the center of the field has three variably sized, pyknotic nuclear fragments. This is a feature of dyserythropoiesis. Canine blood smear; 100× objective.

erative anemia. Macrocytic nonregenerative anemia also has been documented in a cat with folate deficiency. Macrocytosis occurs in some poodles and has little clinical significance. A third feature of dyserythropoiesis is the presence of sideroblasts and siderocytes, which, respectively, are nucleated or anucleated red blood cells with bluish granular material in the cytoplasm. This material is iron and can be difficult to distinguish from the common cause of basophilic stippling, which is RNA accumulation. A Prussian blue stain, or other iron-specific stain, is necessary to confirm that the granular material is iron. Other abnormalities of erythrocytic differentiation that may be present include the presence of cells with multiple nuclei and abnormal nuclear shapes (Fig. 9.12). Abnormal nuclear shapes of erythrocytic precursors have also been seen after the administration of vincristine.

Myelodysplasia of granulocytic development is known as dysgranulopoiesis. Nuclear changes that may be seen include hyper- and hyposegmentation as well as nuclear fragmentation. Changes in the cytoplasm of the cells include decreased numbers of granules or abnormal granule shapes, which can be most easily recognized in eosinophils or basophils. Giant neutrophils may be present also; however, enlarged neutrophils and possibly giant neutrophils may be seen as a sign of neutrophil toxicity during inflammatory disease (Fig. 9.13).

Myelodysplasia of platelet production is known as dysthrombopoiesis. The main feature that may be present in the peripheral blood is a high number of giant platelets (Figs. 9.14 and 9.15). These platelets may be hypo- or hypergranular. In cats, the presence of low to moderate numbers of large platelets is common, irrespective of the underlying disease state.

Acute Myeloid Leukemia

Acute Undifferentiated Leukemia   The most poorly differentiated acute myeloid leukemia is acute undifferentiated leukemia. In this condition, the blood contains high numbers of cells that are very difficult to classify on the basis of their morphology, as well as

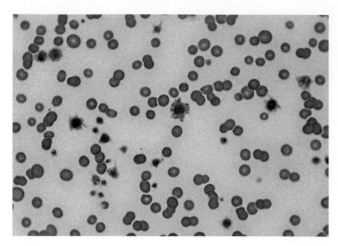

Figure 9.14 Giant platelets. Many giant platelets are present. Because of the high numbers and very large size of the platelets, this represents dysthrombopoiesis. Feline blood smear; 50× objective.

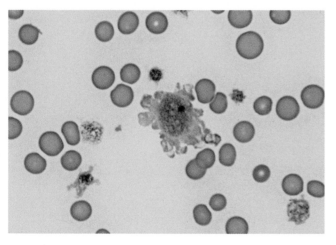

Figure 9.15 Giant platelet. This is a greater magnification of the blood smear shown in Figure 9.13. A very large, abnormally shaped giant platelet is present (center). Feline blood smear; 100× objective.

enzyme cytochemical staining patterns. Included in this category is a disease in cats previously known as reticuloendotheliosis. In this disease, many blasts and immature-appearing cells are present in the circulation, with some of the cells having eccentrically placed round nuclei with moderate amounts of blue cytoplasm either with or without purple granules (Fig. 9.16). The nuclear chromatin may be coarse and similar to cells of the erythrocytic lineage; however, cytoplasmic features are often similar to cells of the granulocytic lineage.

Acute Myeloblastic Leukemia Acute myeloblastic leukemia, also known as acute granulocytic leukemia, has high numbers of immature granulocytic precur-

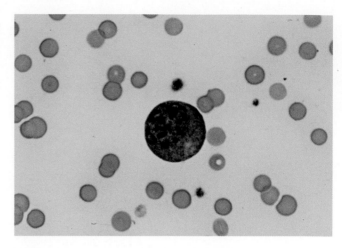

Figure 9.16 Acute undifferentiated leukemia. There is a very large cell (center) with a round to oval, eccentrically placed nucleus; a coarsely granular chromatin pattern; and moderate amounts of deep blue cytoplasm with pink-purple granules. This cell has features of both erythrocytic and granulocytic precursors. Feline blood smear; 100× objective.

sors in the peripheral blood. Typically, myeloblasts, and possibly promyelocytes, are present in high numbers (Figs. 9.17 and 9.18). Other more mature granulocytic cells may be present as well; however, in contrast to severe inflammatory disease, these more differentiated granulocytes are in the minority. If just myeloblasts are present, it can be difficult to distinguish these cells from other blast cells such as lymphoblasts or monoblasts. In these cases, enzyme cytochemical staining or immunophenotyping is essential for accurate classification.

Acute Monocytic Leukemia Acute monocytic leukemia is recognized by the high number of monocytes, as well as monocytic precursors, including promonocytes and monoblasts, in the circulation (Figs. 9.19 and 9.20). Leukemias that just have monoblasts present can be difficult to distinguish from acute myeloblastic leukemia or acute lymphocytic leukemia.

Myelomonocytic Leukemia Myelomonocytic leukemia is a neoplastic proliferation of both types of cells of the granulocytic and monocytic lineage. It has the combined features of both acute myeloblastic leukemia and acute monocytic leukemia.

Erythroleukemia Erythroleukemia, as the name implies, is a leukemia of both red and white cell lineages. Both erythrocytic and leukocytic precursors are present in the circulation (Figs. 9.21 and 9.22). An abnormal number of early precursors are typically present. This condition must be distinguished from a leukoeryth-

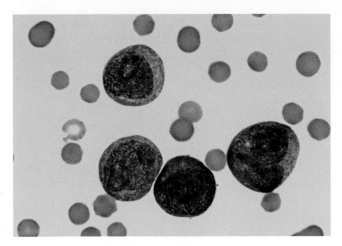

Figure 9.17 Acute myeloblastic (or acute granulocytic) leukemia. Four very large cells are present with round to indented, immature-appearing nuclei. Without cytochemical stains, these cells of the granulocytic lineage are difficult to distinguish from immature cells of the lymphocytic or monocytic lineage. Feline blood smear, from 1985 American Society for Veterinary Clinical Pathology slide review, courtesy of J. T. Blue; 100× objective.

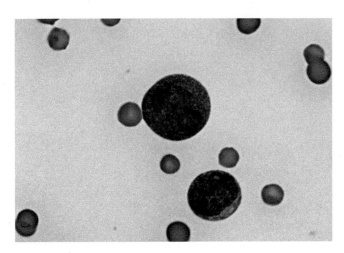

Figure 9.18 Acute myeloblastic leukemia. Another field of view of the blood smear shown in Figure 9.16. The large cell in the center has an oval immature nucleus and pink cytoplasmic granules. The presence of the cytoplasmic granules similar to those of a normal promyelocyte helps to classify this leukemia as granulocytic in origin. The smaller cell in the lower right may be a component of the leukemic process. Feline blood smear, from 1985 American Society for Veterinary Clinical Pathology slide review, courtesy of J. T. Blue; 100× objective.

Figure 9.19 Acute monocytic leukemia. The five cells with deeply indented nuclei and occasionally vacuolated cytoplasm have features similar to normal monocytes. Canine blood smear; 50× objective.

Figure 9.20 Acute monocytic leukemia. Another field of view of the blood smear shown in Figure 9.19. The large cell (center) with an oval nucleus and multiple, poorly distinct nucleoli is a monoblast. Because of the presence of high numbers of cells with monocytic morphology, as shown in Figure 9.19, and monoblasts, this represents acute monocytic leukemia. Cytochemical staining for confirmation of cell lineage is recommended. Canine blood smear; 100× objective.

roblastic state, which is a nonneoplastic process that occurs in times of extreme peripheral demand for red and white cells. The main way to distinguish these two when evaluating the blood smear is that in erythroleukemia, there are typically a disproportionate number of early erythrocytic and leukocytic precursors as compared with the number of mature cells. In contrast, during a leukoerythroblastic response, there are typically more mature erythrocytic and leukocytic precursors present than there are immature cells.

Megakaryoblastic Leukemia Megakaryoblastic leukemia is recognized by the high number of megakaryoblasts in the circulation. As with other poorly differentiated leukemias, the megakaryoblasts may be

Figure 9.21 Erythroleukemia. Three nucleated red blood cells are present in the upper-left corner. A large, immature cell, probably an early granulocytic precursor, is present in the lower-right corner. Feline blood smear; 100× objective.

Figure 9.22 Erythroleukemia. Another field of view of the blood smear shown in Figure 9.21. Cells of the erythrocytic and granulocytic lineage are present. The presence of immature cells of the granulocytic and erythrocytic lineage, the decreased red blood cell density (anemia), and the lack of polychromatophils and mature, segmented neutrophils are representative of erythroleukemia. Feline blood smear; 100× objective.

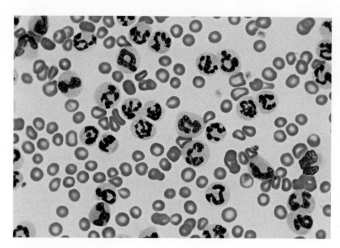

Figure 9.23 Chronic granulocytic leukemia. Many segmented neutrophils are present. The high numbers of neutrophils with a lack of inflammation present in this animal are diagnostic of chronic granulocytic leukemia. Canine blood smear; 50× objective.

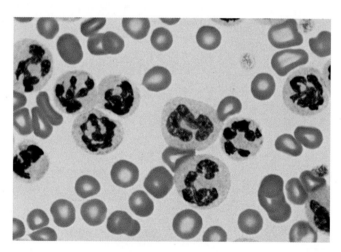

Figure 9.24 Chronic granulocytic leukemia. This is a greater magnification of the blood smear shown in Figure 9.23. Note the many segmented neutrophils present, the majority of which are hypersegmented. Canine blood smear; 100× objective.

difficult to differentiate from other blast cells on the basis of morphology alone. Increases and decreases in platelet numbers, as well as the presence of giant platelets and hypo- and hypergranulation of the platelets, have also been documented.

Chronic Myeloid Leukemia

Chronic myeloid leukemia is recognized by high numbers of well-differentiated cells of the granulocytic lineage (neutrophilic, eosinophilic, or basophilic).

These disorders are named by the predominant cell type present in the blood. For example, if mainly eosinophils are present, it is an eosinophilic leukemia. In these cases, as well as other chronic myeloid leukemias, in addition to the presence of mature cells, immature cells may also be present. This can be seen in eosinophilic leukemia, whereby eosinophilic bands, metamyelocytes, and myelocytes may be present; however, the mature cell type vastly predominates. If cells of the neutrophilic lineage predominate, the disorder is known as chronic granulocytic or myelocytic leukemia (Figs. 9.23 and 9.24).

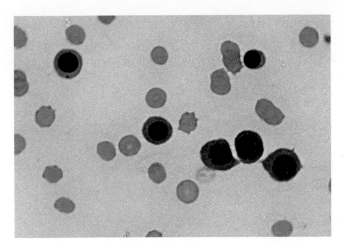

Figure 9.25 Erythremic myelosis. Six nucleated red blood cells are present. This finding, associated with low red cell density (anemia) and a lack of polychromasia, is supportive of erythremic myelosis. Feline blood smear; 100× objective.

Figure 9.26 Marked thrombocytosis. Many platelets are present throughout the field. This extreme thrombocytosis is typical of essential thrombocythemia. Canine blood smear, from 1987 American Society for Veterinary Clinical Pathology slide review, courtesy of J. G. Zinkl; 100× objective.

Others

Erythremic Myelosis   Erythremic myelosis has historically been classified as a leukemia of the erythrocytic lineage. This disorder has recently been renamed as either myelodysplastic syndrome with erythroid predominance or erythroleukemia with erythroid predominance; it mainly occurs in cats. In this disorder, erythrocytic precursors are present in the blood with a lack of significant numbers of polychromatophils (Fig. 9.25). Most of the cells are usually metarubricytes and rubricytes, but prorubricytes and rubriblasts may be present also.

Polycythemia Vera   A well-differentiated leukemia of the erythrocytic lineage is known as polycythemia vera, in which there are very high numbers of morphologically normal erythrocytes. Rarely, there have been reports of increased numbers of white blood cells in these animals as well. These findings suggest a multiple cell lineage effect, rather than a sole erythrocytic abnormality.

Essential Thrombocythemia   A well-differentiated leukemia of the megakaryocytic lineage is known as essential thrombocythemia (Fig. 9.26). Abnormal platelet morphology such as giant platelets and hypo- and hypergranulation of the platelets has been documented in addition to the marked thrombocytosis that is seen.

Neoplastic Proliferation of Mast Cells   Although not a true leukemia, neoplastic proliferation of mast cells may occur in the bone marrow, with subsequent release of these cells into circulation (Figs. 9.27 and 9.28). This can result in often finding high numbers of poorly to well-granulated mast cells in the circulation. Mast cells present in the circulation (mastocytemia) secondary to a neoplastic proliferation must be differentiated from mast cells in the circulation in association with inflammatory disease. Typically, when mast cells are found in the circulation secondary to inflammatory disease, the cells are well granulated and present in very low numbers. This, also, often is a very transient response.

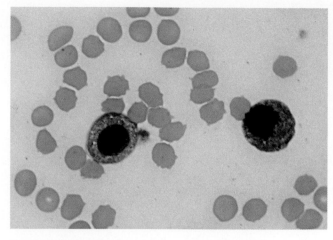

Figure 9.27 Mastocytemia. Three mast cells are present. If there is a large number of mast cells present in the circulation and inflammatory disease is not present, a systemic mast cell neoplastic process is likely. Feline blood smear; 50× objective.

Figure 9.28 Mastocytemia. Another field from the blood smear shown in Figure 9.27. Two well-granulated mast cells are present. Feline blood smear; 100× objective.

CHAPTER TEN
MISCELLANEOUS FINDINGS

There are several different cell types that are often not classified accurately by the inexperienced hematologist. These cell types are contrasted here. Small lymphocytes are sometimes confused with nucleated red blood cells, specifically, rubricytes (Fig. 10.1). Both of these cells have very high nuclear to cytoplasmic ratios and round nuclei. The main difference is the chromatin pattern of the nuclei. Small lymphocytes have a homogeneous, glassy- to smudged-appearing nuclear chromatin with some areas of condensation. In contrast, rubricytes have a much more coarsely granular and clumped nuclear chromatin. The color of the cytoplasm may also be helpful. The cytoplasm of the rubricyte ranges from deep blue to reddish-blue, whereas the cytoplasm of the small lymphocyte is typically light blue but may be deep blue if reactive.

Large lymphocytes are sometimes confused with monocytes, which do not have vacuoles in the cytoplasm (Fig. 10.2). Both cells have a moderate nuclear-to-cytoplasmic ratio. Large lymphocyte nuclei are typically round to oval but may be indented. In con-

trast, monocyte nuclei may be round to oval but usually have multiple indentations. The chromatin pattern of the large lymphocyte is more homogeneous than the netlike chromatin with several clumped areas of the monocyte. Both cells have blue cytoplasm; however, the cytoplasm of the monocyte is typically blue-gray. If a large cell that may be a monocyte or lymphocyte is observed, it may be useful to find a more classic monocyte with vacuoles and to compare this cell with the cell in question and see whether the nuclear chromatin and color of the cytoplasm are similar or different.

Monocytes also are sometimes confused with toxic band neutrophils and metamyelocytes. Differentiating these cells is one of the great challenges in cell identification (Fig. 10.3). Monocytes, toxic band neutrophils, and metamyelocytes are often of similar size with blue cytoplasm. The nucleus of the monocyte can be band- or kidney bean–shaped, similar to the nucleus of the band neutrophil and metamyelocyte, respectively. One of the primary differences among these three cell types is related to the nuclear chromatin

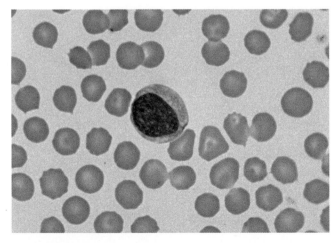

Figure 10.1 Rubricyte versus lymphocyte. The cell (left of center) with a round nucleus and with very clumped chromatin and rim of reddish-blue cytoplasm is a rubricyte. The cell (right of center) with a round to oval, slightly indented nucleus and smudged nuclear chromatin with some areas of condensation is a small lymphocyte. Note that the cytoplasm of the lymphocyte is light blue compared with the reddish-blue cytoplasm of the rubricyte. Canine blood smear; 100× objective.

Figure 10.2 Large lymphocyte. The cell with the oval nucleus and moderate amount of light blue cytoplasm is a large lymphocyte. Note that the chromatin is more homogeneous compared with the netlike chromatin with areas of condensation of the monocytes in Figure 10.3. Canine blood smear; 100× objective.

Figure 10.3 Monocyte versus toxic band neutrophil. The two nucleated cells in the lower-left quadrant are monocytes; the large nucleated cell in the upper-right quadrant is a toxic band neutrophil. Note that the chromatin pattern of the band neutrophil is much more condensed, or clumped, compared with the more open, netlike chromatin pattern of the monocyte. Canine blood smear; 100× objective.

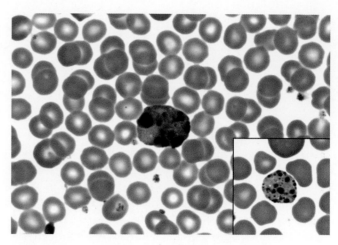

Figure 10.5 Karyorrhexis. The cell in the center is a white blood cell undergoing necrosis with the beginning fragmentation of the nucleus (karyorrhexis). The inset (lower right) is from the same blood smear and demonstrates karyorrhexis with more numerous nuclear fragments. Rat blood smear; 100× objective.

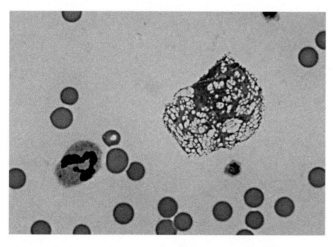

Figure 10.4 Smudge cell. The large, light purple, netlike structure in the right center of the field is a broken, or smudge, cell; this is free nuclear chromatin material. There is a neutrophil present (lower left). Feline blood smear; 100× objective.

Figure 10.6 Pyknotic cell. The cell (center) with pink cytoplasm and four markedly condensed nuclear fragments is a pyknotic neutrophil. There is a normal segmented neutrophil present to the right of the pyknotic neutrophil. Canine blood smear; 100× objective.

patterns. The monocyte nuclear chromatin is lacy or netlike, with some areas of condensation, and the chromatin of the cells of the neutrophilic lineage is more condensed or clumped. The presence of Döhle bodies is also helpful in accurately identifying the cell as an immature neutrophil; Döhle bodies are not present in monocytes.

Other miscellaneous cell types include smudge, pyknotic, mitotic, and necrotic cells. Smudge cells are just broken cells (Fig. 10.4), and it is impossible to accurately identify their exact origin. Typically,

however, they will not have intact cell membranes, and the cytoplasm is lost; only free nuclear chromatin material is present. These cells are sometimes also called basket cells because of the delicate, woven, basket-like strands of dispersed nuclear chromatin. Low numbers of these cells may be present in normal preparations. High numbers of broken cells may be present if the blood sample is lipemic or, sometimes, when high numbers of neoplastic and possibly more-fragile cells are present.

Cells that are undergoing necrosis are difficult to identify. Karyorrhexis is a fragmentation of the nucleus of the cell undergoing degeneration (Fig. 10.5). Cells

Figure 10.7 Mitotic figure. The blue cell with an irregularly shaped nucleus is a cell undergoing mitosis. Canine blood smear; 100× objective.

Figure 10.8 Mature red blood cells and polychromatophils. The bluish-purple cells in the center of the field and upper-left corner are polychromatophils. The other cells are mature red blood cells and platelets. Bovine blood smear; Diff-Quik stain; 100× objective.

that are undergoing pyknosis have very condensed nuclear chromatin (Fig. 10.6), and it is often impossible to identify the cell of origin.

Mitotic cells are cells that are dividing, and thus the chromosomes are visible (Fig. 10.7). The exact origin of the mitotic cells is often impossible to identify. It is uncommon to see these in the peripheral blood, but if they are present in significant numbers, a neoplastic process may be present.

Cell identification often depends on recognizing the color of the cell, which in turn depends on the type and quality of the stain used. A commonly used, rapid, modified Wright's stain is Diff-Quik. With this stain, the color of the blood cells is slightly different compared with the color of the cells in the photomicrographs shown throughout the text, which are Wright's stained. One of the major color differences is that of the red blood cells. Often, the mature red blood cells stain bluish-gray to brownish-red with Diff-Quik (Fig. 10.8). Polychromatophils may be difficult to identify because they stain bluish-red to bluish-purple. The cytoplasm of the neutrophils, also, is often bluer, which may be confused with mild toxicity. Finally, the chromatin pattern of most of the nucleated cells is often more accentuated or clumped when Diff-Quik stain is used (Fig. 10.9).

Two extracellular organisms that may be present in the blood are microfilaria and trypanosomes. Microfilaria are easily recognized, based on their very large size. Typically, they are a few hundred microns long and several microns thick (Fig. 10.10). Because of their large size, the organisms often end up on the feathered edge of the blood smear. The two most commonly recognized microfilaria are *Dirofilaria immitis* and

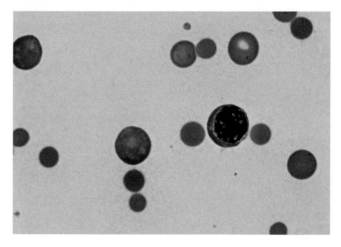

Figure 10.9 Rubricyte. The cell in the right center of the field is a rubricyte. Note the marked clumped chromatin compared with the rubricyte shown in Figure 10.1. Polychromatophils (larger and bluish-purple–staining cells) and mature red blood cells are present also. Bovine blood smear; Diff-Quik stain; 100× objective.

Dipetalonema reconditum, which are most often found in dogs. Several characteristics, including length, shape, and thickness, can be used to distinguish these two different types of microfilaria. These features are best evaluated in wet mounts or fixed preparations. In general, if microfilaria are present on an air-dried blood smear, they are reported as just microfilaria, and other tests are necessary for accurate classification. Trypanosomes are rarely seen in the peripheral blood of animals, but their significance varies from

Figure 10.10 Microfilaria. The very large, elongated structure in the center of the field is a microfilaria. Canine blood smear; 50× objective.

Figure 10.11 *Trypanosoma theileri.* The ribbon-like structure with tapered ends is typical of trypanosome species. This specimen is surrounded by a clump of platelets. Notice the faintly staining membrane along the convex border and the elongate, delicate flagellum at one end. Bovine blood smear; 100× objective.

area to area. Of the widely distributed nonpathogenic species, *Trypanosoma theileri* in cattle (Fig. 10.11) in North America, Western Europe, and Australia, and *T. melophagium* in sheep, are the most common. Pathogenic trypanosomes are important parasites and may be found in horses and cattle in tropical and subtropical zones. *Trypanosoma cruzi* in dogs is mainly found in the United States and South and Central America. These are large, elongated, ribbon-like structures, often with tapered ends. They frequently have an indistinct, undulating membrane on one side and a small, round, deeply staining internal structure known as a kinetoplast. *T. theileri* are 25–120 µm long. *T. cruzi* are 16–20 µm long.

CHAPTER ELEVEN
AVIAN HEMATOLOGY

GENERAL FEATURES

Avian blood cell morphology is very similar to reptilian blood cell morphology. Avian granulocytes (heterophil, eosinophil, basophil) differ the most from those of mammals; however, avian lymphocytes and monocytes are similar, morphologically, to those of mammals. Like reptiles, birds also have nucleated red blood cells. Despite the differences, correct identification of all avian leukocytes and other cells is simple and will depend on having good baseline knowledge of the species most frequently seen, prompt processing of the blood sample, and good, consistent staining technique and supplies. Acceptable samples to prepare blood smears include fresh blood (no anticoagulant) and blood mixed with anticoagulants (heparin, EDTA, or sodium citrate). EDTA may cause destruction of red blood cells in some bird species and therefore may be unsuitable in some instances. To improve one's ability to correctly identify all avian leukocytes, it is imperative that students frequently examine blood smears from healthy and diseased birds, particularly the species that are most commonly seen. As is the case for all blood smears, it is important to prevent formalin fumes or formalin liquid from contacting unstained smears because formalin will negatively affect the staining quality of the smears.

NORMAL RED BLOOD CELL MORPHOLOGY

In health, mature red blood cells are elliptical cells with round to oval nuclei and darkly staining nuclear chromatin (Fig. 11.1). The cytoplasm stains homogeneously pink to orange-red because of hemoglobin. The color of red blood cells will vary with the type and quality of the staining method. Low numbers of polychromatophils (< 5 percent) may occur in healthy birds and are characterized by a pale blue color of the cytoplasm of the red blood cell (Fig. 11.2). Anisocytosis and poikilocytosis are typically minimal in blood from normal birds.

Figure 11.1 Normal avian red blood cells. Elliptical cells with round to oval nuclei and darkly staining nuclear chromatin are red blood cells. The lower image was from a quick-stained blood smear and contains a mature heterophil and two thrombocytes in the mid- to bottom left of the field; the upper image was from a Wright's stained blood smear. Goose (unspecified genus, top image) and cockatiel (*Nymphicus hollandicus*, bottom image) blood smears; 100× objective.

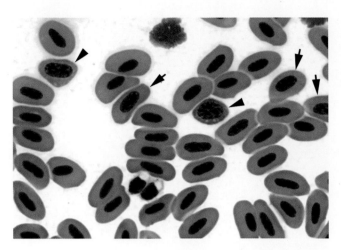

Figure 11.2 Red blood cell precursors. Polychromatophils (arrows) and less mature red blood cell precursors (arrowheads) have bluish cytoplasm and nuclear chromatin that is not as dense and dark as mature red blood cells. The nucleus of less mature red blood cell precursors is less oval than that of mature red blood cells. The two nucleated cells in the bottom of the field are thrombocytes. Cockatiel (*Nymphicus hollandicus*) blood smear; 100× objective.

Figure 11.4 Basophilic stippling. Basophilic stippling is present in the two red blood cells in the upper and lower center of the field. The clear cytoplasmic areas in the red blood cell in the top center are an artifact. A heterophil is on the center right of the field. The inset is a greater magnification of a red blood cell with basophilic stippling from the same blood smear. Clear cytoplasmic areas are an artifact. Duck (unspecified genus) blood smear; 100× objective.

Figure 11.3 Red blood cell precursors. The many oval nucleated cells with bluish cytoplasm are polychromatophils or less mature red blood cell precursors. There are only a few mature red blood cells in the field (orange staining cytoplasm). The inset contains a greater magnification of a binucleated red blood cell precursor from the same blood smear. Parrot (unspecified genus) blood smear; 100× objective.

Figure 11.5 Pyknosis. The red blood cells (center of the field and in the inset) with densely dark and fragmented nuclei are pyknotic cells. Parrot (unspecified genus); 100× objective.

VARIATIONS IN RED BLOOD CELL MORPHOLOGY

Red blood cell morphologic abnormalities in birds include increased anisocytosis and poikilocytosis, increased numbers of polychromatophils or more immature red blood cell precursors (Figs. 11.2 and 11.3), basophilic stippling (pinpoint blue granules in the cytoplasm; Fig. 11.4), binucleation (Fig. 11.3), pyknosis (Fig. 11.5), or mitoses. These changes may be seen in markedly regenerative responses or with bone marrow disorders. Hypochromasia may occur with iron deficiency, agglutination may occur with immune-mediated processes, and basophilic stippling may occur infrequently with lead intoxication or regenerative responses. Intracytoplasmic inclusions may be caused by protozoal organisms such as *Haemoproteus*

Figure 11.6 *Haemoproteus* sp. The three red blood cells in the center of the field contain elongate ("banana-shaped") intracytoplasmic pink to bluish organisms with dark brown granules that are gametocytes of *Haemoproteus* sp. The oval nucleus of the red blood cells is in the center of the infected cells. The inset is a greater magnification. Pigeon (*Columba livia*) blood smear; quick stain; 100× objective.

Figure 11.8 Heterophils. The cell in the center of the field (upper and lower images) with a lobulated nucleus and elongate red cytoplasmic granules is a mature heterophil. The lower image was from a blood smear of the same bird and was stained with a quick stain; the upper image was from a blood smear stained with Wright's stain. Insets are greater magnifications. Cockatiel (*Nymphicus hollandicus*) blood smears; 100× objective.

NORMAL WHITE BLOOD CELL MORPHOLOGY

Heterophil

In health, the heterophil is generally the most common peripheral blood leukocyte of birds. The mature heterophil nucleus has two to three lobes and is not as lobulated as the nuclei of mature mammalian neutrophils. The heterophil of birds has cytoplasm that is densely packed with elongate, rod- to spindle-shaped, orange to red-brown granules that may partially obscure the nucleus (Plate 3 [p. 83]; Figs. 11.8–11.10). Granules may be round to oval in some species of birds. Quick staining methods may sometimes make the granules of heterophils less distinct (Fig. 11.10).

Figure 11.7 *Leukocytozoon* sp. The bluish oval structure at the upper center of the field with thin pale elongate ends is a nucleated blood cell with a gametocyte of *Leukocytozoon* sp. The curved narrow purple rim adjacent to the parasite is the host cell nucleus. Owl (unspecified genus) blood smear; 100× objective.

sp., *Plasmodium* sp., and *Leukocytozoon* sp. *Haemoproteus* sp. are typically nonpathogenic and do not greatly distort the morphology of red blood cells (Fig. 11.6); however, *Plasmodium* and *Leukocytozoon* sp. (Fig. 11.7) are pathogenic.

Figure 11.9 Heterophil. The cell in the center of the field with a lobulated nucleus and elongate red cytoplasmic granules is a mature heterophil. Pink-headed fruit dove (*Ptilinopus porphyreus*) blood smear; 100× objective.

Figure 11.11 Small lymphocytes. The two cells with a round to slightly oval nucleus, coarsely clumped chromatin, and small amounts of blue cytoplasm are small lymphocytes. Parrot (unspecified genus) blood smear; 100× objective.

Figure 11.10 Heterophil. The cell in the center of the field with a lobulated nucleus and red-orange indistinct cytoplasmic granules is a mature heterophil. Quick stains sometimes will make heterophil granules less distinct than with Wright's stain. Dove (unspecified genus) blood smear; quick stain; 100× objective.

Heterophils from chickens and turkeys are approximately 13 μm in diameter.

Lymphocyte

In health, the lymphocyte is morphologically similar to that of mammals. In general, the lymphocyte has a single, eccentrically located, round nucleus; low to scant amounts of pale blue cytoplasm; and high nuclear to cytoplasmic ratio (Plate 3; Figs. 11.11–11.15). The chromatin is coarsely clumped. Healthy birds have small and larger-sized lymphocytes. Small lymphocytes are typically smaller than heterophils. Other peripheral blood cells that may be confused at times

with lymphocytes include thrombocytes (platelets; Fig. 11.13 and 11.14) and immature red blood cells (Fig. 11.15). Thrombocytes are generally oval rather than round in shape, have very pale blue to nonstaining cytoplasm, and readily clump in blood smears. Immature red blood cells that are round in shape may be confused with lymphocytes; however, lymphocytes have an eccentrically located nucleus versus the typical centrally located nucleus of the immature red blood cells, and lymphocytes generally have a higher nuclear-to-cytoplasmic ratio (i.e., lower amounts of cytoplasm relative to the size of the nucleus). The chromatin pattern of the immature red blood cells will be more similar to that of red blood cells (including polychromatophils) in the same smear. Significantly increased numbers of polychromatophils should increase awareness that round, immature red blood cells may be present in the smear.

Monocyte

The monocyte of birds is similar to that of domestic animals. Monocytes are large mononuclear cells with abundant amounts of blue cytoplasm (Plate 3; Figs. 11.16–11.18). Nuclei are oval to round, sometimes indented or U-shaped. Monocytes are typically larger and have less condensation of the chromatin than lymphocytes. Monocytes from chickens and turkeys are approximately 14 μm in diameter.

Eosinophil

Eosinophils have pale blue cytoplasm that contains numerous round, bright red to pink cytoplasmic

Figure 11.12 Lymphocytes. The two round cells (left top and right bottom of the field) with round nucleus and small to scant amounts of blue cytoplasm are lymphocytes. The variation in the size of lymphocytes, as shown in the image, is normal for birds. Great horned owl (*Bubo virginianus*) blood smear; 100× objective.

Figure 11.14 Small lymphocyte and thrombocyte. The small round cell with a round minimally indented nucleus and scant amounts of blue cytoplasm (center left of field) is a small lymphocyte, and the small oval nucleated cell with low amounts of nearly colorless cytoplasm is a thrombocyte (center right of field). The inset is a greater magnification. Goose (unspecified genus) blood smear; 100× objective.

Figure 11.13 Small lymphocyte and thrombocytes. The round cell with a round to slightly oval nucleus and low amounts of blue cytoplasm (bottom left of field) is a small lymphocyte. The smaller individual to aggregated nucleated oval cells with scant amounts of pale blue cytoplasm are thrombocytes. Cockatiel (*Nymphicus hollandicus*) blood smear; 100× objective.

Figure 11.15 Small lymphocytes and red blood cell precursors. Two small lymphocytes (arrows) and multiple red blood cell precursors are shown. One of the lymphocytes has cytoplasmic vacuoles. Most of the red blood cell precursors are polychromatophils; however, there is a round, more immature red blood cell in the lower center right of the field. Parrot (unspecified genus) blood smear; 100× objective.

granules (Plate 3; Figs. 11.19–11.21). Sometimes, depending on the bird species and the staining method, eosinophil granules will be pale blue to blue-green in color (Plate 3; Figs. 11.19 and 11.20). Eosinophils may be differentiated from heterophils by the shape (generally round in eosinophils) and color (more intensely pink to red in eosinophils from most birds) of the granules. Other characteristics

that may be of help are that the numbers of eosinophils are typically less than that of heterophils, the chromatin may be denser or darker staining than that of heterophils, or the cytoplasm of the eosinophil is pale blue versus the generally colorless cytoplasm of the heterophil. Eosinophils from chickens and turkeys are approximately 12 μm in diameter.

Figure 11.16 Monocyte. The nucleated cell with an indented nucleus and blue cytoplasm is a monocyte. Cockatiel (*Nymphicus hollandicus*) blood smear; 100× objective.

Figure 11.17 Monocyte. The oval nucleated cell with an indented nucleus and blue cytoplasm is a monocyte. Parrot (unspecified genus) blood smear; quick stain; 100× objective.

Figure 11.18 Monocyte. The nucleated cell with an indented, U-shaped nucleus and blue cytoplasm is a monocyte. A thrombocyte (center left of the field) and a mature heterophil (top right of the field) are also shown. Dove (unspecified genus); quick stain; 100× objective.

Figure 11.19 Eosinophils and heterophil. The cell with a lobulated nucleus and round pink to red cytoplasmic granules (upper image, bottom center of field; lower image, center of field) is an eosinophil. The cell with red elongate granules is a mature heterophil (upper image, top center of field). Insets are greater magnification images of the eosinophils. The lower image was from a blood smear of the same bird and was stained with a quick stain; the upper image was from a blood smear stained with Wright's stain. Cockatiel (*Nymphicus hollandicus*) blood smear; 100× objective.

Figure 11.20 Eosinophil. The cell with a lobulated nucleus and round bluish cytoplasmic granules is an eosinophil. Parrot (unspecified genus) blood smear; 100× objective.

Figure 11.21 Eosinophil and heterophil. The cell with a lobulated nucleus, pale blue cytoplasm, and round orange-red cytoplasmic granules (left center of field) is an eosinophil. The cell with red indistinct cytoplasmic granules is a mature heterophil (right center of field). Inset is a greater magnification of the eosinophil. Mute swan (*Cygnus olor*) blood smear; 100× objective.

Figure 11.23 Basophil. The cell with a round nucleus and dark purple granules is a basophil (left center of the field). Inset is a greater magnification of the basophil. Parrot (unspecified genus) blood smear; 100× objective.

Figure 11.22 Basophil and eosinophil. The cell with a lobulated nucleus and dark purple granules is a basophil (lower left of field). The cell with a lobulated nucleus and round pink to red cytoplasmic granules is an eosinophil (upper right of field). Inset is a greater magnification of the basophil. Cockatiel (*Nymphicus hollandicus*) blood smear; 100× objective.

Basophil

Basophils have numerous small, round, dark purple cytoplasmic granules (Plate 3; Figs. 11.22 and 11.23). The granules may be so numerous as to obscure the nucleus. A difference from the mammalian basophil is that the nucleus of the basophil in birds is generally round to oval and not lobulated like in mammals. The cytoplasm of avian basophils is sometimes vacuolated

or foamy; however, a few granules will still remain and may be easier to locate over the nucleus (Plate 3).

VARIATIONS IN WHITE CELL MORPHOLOGY

Granulocytes

The range of granulocytic leukocyte morphologic abnormalities that can occur in birds in response to inflammatory and noninflammatory conditions is similar to that of mammals and includes heterophil left shift, heterophil toxicity, and giant heterophils (Figs. 11.24–11.26). Similar to domestic animal species, left shift refers to the presence of immature heterophil precursors in the peripheral blood in response to an inflammatory insult that overwhelms the capacity of the bone marrow to respond. Left shifts may consist of band heterophils, metamyelocytes, or more immature precursors (Figs. 11.24 and 11.26). Band heterophils have a nonlobulated, U-shaped nucleus and cytoplasmic contents that are similar to mature heterophils. More immature precursors may have round to oval nuclei, darker blue cytoplasm, and a mixture of rod-shaped granules and rounder granules. A few granules may be blue to purple. Heterophil toxicity typically manifests as darker blue cytoplasm, cytoplasmic foaminess, or vacuolation and may be accompanied by morphologic changes in the granules consisting of round shape or blue- to purple-colored granules side by side with the typical heterophil gran-

Figure 11.24 Heterophil toxicity and left shift. The three cells (center of field) with cytoplasmic vacuoles, indistinct red cytoplasmic granules, and decreased nuclear lobulation or with round to oval nuclei are toxic and immature (left-shift) heterophils. There are also numerous polychromatophils and other oval to round, more immature red blood cell precursors in the field. The inset is a greater magnification of an immature heterophil (left) and a mature heterophil (right) from the same blood smear. Parrot (unspecified genus) blood smear; 100× objective.

Figure 11.25 Heterophil toxicity. The cell with a lobulated nucleus and round orange-red to purple, variably sized granules is a toxic heterophil (upper image, center of field). The cell with a lobulated nucleus and oval orange-red granules is a mature heterophil (lower image, center of field). The insets are greater magnifications of the heterophils. Goose (unspecified genus) blood smear; 100× objective.

ules (Figs. 11.25 and 11.26). Increased numbers of Döhle bodies, as occurs in mammals, is not a common finding during inflammation in birds. Giant heterophils may occur with inflammation and manifests as larger-than-normal heterophils. Degranulation of granulocytes can also occur and results in clear, distinct vacuoles in the cytoplasm of heterophils or other granulocytes. Pyknotic leukocytes may occur in the peripheral blood.

Lymphocytes and Monocytes

Similar to in mammals, reactive lymphocytes, plasma cells, and atypical/leukemic cells may occur in birds. Reactive lymphocytes have increased amounts of darker blue cytoplasm, increased density of the nucleus, and may have a small perinuclear clear zone (Fig. 11.27). Lymphocytes with small pink granules may occur in low numbers in healthy birds. Plasma cells may occur rarely and have abundant amounts of blue cytoplasm, prominent perinuclear clear zones, and dense, eccentrically located nucleus. Atypical mononuclear cells (lymphocytic or monocytic) may occur with leukemia. Leukemic diseases are uncommon in pet birds.

Figure 11.26 Heterophil toxicity and left shift. The cell with a round nucleus, numerous purple to orange round granules, and small amounts of cytoplasmic vacuolation is an immature and toxic heterophil. The inset is a greater magnification. Goose (unspecified genus) blood smear; 100× objective.

WHITE BLOOD CELL INCLUSIONS AND PARASITES

Inclusions in avian leukocytes are relatively infrequent findings. Inclusions are typically of infectious origin. Parasites include *Atoxoplasma* sp. in lymphocytes of passerine birds (includes perching songbirds).

Figure 11.27 Reactive lymphocyte and thrombocytes. The round cell with a round, minimally indented nucleus and dark blue cytoplasm is a reactive lymphocyte (left of field). The nucleus of the cell has a few dense dark aggregates of chromatin. A cluster of thrombocytes is present in the lower left of the field, and a normal small lymphocyte is in the upper right of the field. The inset is a greater magnification of the reactive lymphocyte. Parrot (unspecified genus) blood smear; 100× objective.

Figure 11.29 Thrombocytes. The clustered or individual small nucleated oval cells with colorless to pale blue cytoplasm (center right and center left of field) are thrombocytes. One of the thrombocytes has a small pink granule. The inset is a greater magnification of two thrombocytes. Goose (unspecified genus) blood smear; 100× objective.

Noninfectious causes of inclusions in leukocytes are uncommon.

THROMBOCYTE MORPHOLOGY IN HEALTH AND DISEASE

Avian thrombocytes are generally oval nucleated cells with colorless to pale blue cytoplasm and condensed round to oval nucleus (Figs. 11.27–11.29). Sometimes thrombocytes have a round shape in some blood smears and the cytoplasm may contain a single to a few small vacuoles or pink granules (Fig. 11.30). Thrombocytes may be confused with small lympho-

Figure 11.28 Thrombocytes. The clustered nucleated oval cells with low to scant amounts of colorless to pale blue cytoplasm (upper image, center of field) or pale pink cytoplasm (lower image, top and bottom center of field) are thrombocytes. The lower image was from a blood smear of the same bird and was stained with a quick stain; the upper image was from a blood smear stained with Wright's stain. The insets are greater magnifications of the thrombocytes. Cockatiel (*Nymphicus hollandicus*) blood smear; 100× objective.

cytes but can be differentiated from lymphocytes on the basis of the typical oval shape of the thrombocyte versus the round shape of the lymphocyte, the generally colorless to pale staining cytoplasm of the thrombocytes, and the tendency of thrombocytes to clump in blood smears. Inclusions may rarely occur within thrombocytes and may be caused by protozoa such as *Plasmodium* sp.

EXTRACELLULAR BLOOD PARASITES

Microfilaria (Fig. 11.31), bacteria, and protozoa may occur in birds, particularly wild-caught pet birds from other localities and local wildlife.

Figure 11.30 Granulation in thrombocytes. The round nucleated cells with pale blue cytoplasm and pinpoint pink to magenta granules are thrombocytes (center of the field). There is a small lymphocyte (arrowhead), two red blood cells with basophilic stippling (arrows), and a mature heterophil (top left of field). The inset is a greater magnification of several thrombocytes. Duck (unspecified genus) blood smear; 100× objective.

Figure 11.31 Microfilaria. The elongate serpentine extracellular organism in the center of the field is a microfilaria. Owl (unspecified genus) blood smear; quick stain; 100× objective.

PLATE 3. Overview diagram of leukocytes in healthy birds. Heterophils typically have red to orange elongate cytoplasmic granules and a lobulated nucleus. The granules may be so numerous that it may be difficult to see individual granules. Lymphocytes and monocytes are similar to those of domestic animals. Lymphocytes have scant to low amounts of blue cytoplasm and may be small in size (bottom lymphocyte in the diagram) or slightly larger (top lymphocyte in the diagram). Monocytes have abundant blue cytoplasm and an oval to indented nucleus. Eosinophils generally have lobulated nuclei and round cytoplasmic granules. In some bird species, the granules are pink to pale red, and in other bird species, the granules may have a blue to green hue. Basophils will have oval to mildly lobulated nuclei with dark purple granules. Basophils may sometimes appear vacuolated.

| Heterophils | Lymphocytes | Monocytes | Eosinophils | Basophils |

CHAPTER TWELVE
REPTILIAN HEMATOLOGY

GENERAL FEATURES

Reptilian blood cell morphology, especially that of reptilian granulocytes (heterophil, eosinophil, and basophil) and red blood cells, differs the most from those of mammals. Despite the differences, correct identification of all reptilian cells is simple but will depend on prompt processing of blood samples, and good, consistent staining technique and supplies (Fig. 12.1). Inadvertent overstaining may result in inappropriate color characteristics of the blood cells (Fig. 12.1). The best sample with which to prepare blood smears is fresh blood (no anticoagulant), but blood mixed with anticoagulant can also be used if the smear is made promptly after blood collection. EDTA is considered an acceptable anticoagulant for use in some lizards; however, EDTA may cause destruction of red blood cells in other reptiles, such as chelonians (turtles and tortoises). For this reason and because plasma can be harvested for clinical chemistry evaluation, heparin is generally considered a good choice for use in reptiles. Drawbacks to the use of heparin include clumping of thrombocytes and leukocytes, the occurrence of a blue staining background in blood smears, and possible interference with determination of sodium in plasma if sodium heparin is used as an anticoagulant. To improve one's ability to correctly identify all reptil-

ian cells, it is imperative to frequently examine blood smears from healthy and diseased reptiles, particularly the species that are most commonly seen in practice. It is also important to prevent formalin fumes or formalin liquid from contacting unstained smears because formalin will negatively affect the staining quality of the smears.

NORMAL RED BLOOD CELL MORPHOLOGY

Reptilian red blood cells are significantly different from those of most domestic animals. In health, mature red blood cells are elliptical cells with round to oval nuclei, smooth to minimally irregular nuclear membranes, and darkly staining nuclear chromatin (Fig. 12.2). Their size varies greatly according to the species of reptile but can range in size from approximately 13 to 25 μm in their greatest dimension. With some exceptions, turtle red blood cells are generally larger, and lizard red blood cells, for example those of *Lacerta* sp., are generally smaller. Nuclear-to-cytoplasmic ratios also vary between reptilian species. The cytoplasm stains homogeneously pink to orange-red because of hemoglobin. However, the cytoplasm may appear green-blue when overstained with some quick stains

Figure 12.1 Comparison of staining characteristics with different staining methods. (A) Overstaining with a quick stain. (B) Blood smear from the same iguana as in panel A but stained with Wright's stain. Notice the difference in the color of the cytoplasm of red blood cells and of the heterophil granules. (C) Blood smear from an iguana stained with a quick stain but not overstained. The colors match the expected coloration of reptilian blood cells. (D) Blood smear from the same iguana as image C but stained with Wright's stain. Green iguana (*Iguana iguana*) blood smears; 100× objective.

**Snake
mature
red blood cell**

**Lizard
mature
red blood cell**

**Lizard
polychromatophil**

Figure 12.2 Reptilian red blood cells. Normal red blood cells from a snake and a lizard. Sometimes red blood cells have small bluish inclusions in the cytoplasm, as shown in the snake red blood cell. Compared with mature red blood cells, the polychromatophil has blue cytoplasm and a larger, less darkly staining nucleus. Snake (*Boa constrictor*) and green iguana (*Iguana iguana*) blood smears; 100× objective.

Figure 12.3 Red blood cells and red blood cell precursors. A polychromatophil (bottom center of the field), and three less mature round red blood cell precursors (left, top, and right of the field) are shown. The round, less mature, red blood cells have irregular nuclear margins, coarsely clumped chromatin, and dark blue cytoplasm. The small dots throughout the image are artifacts (dust particles). Red blood cell neoplasia was suspected in this animal. Green iguana (*Iguana iguana*) blood smear; quick stain; 100× objective.

(Fig. 12.1) or blue when exposed to formalin. Some species of reptiles may have generally single, small, homogeneous, blue, round cytoplasmic inclusions in red blood cells of healthy individuals (Fig. 12.2). These inclusions must be differentiated from infectious organisms and may be degenerate organelles or artifacts. Low numbers of polychromatophils may occur in healthy reptiles (Fig. 12.2), particularly those that are shedding.

VARIATIONS IN RED BLOOD CELL MORPHOLOGY

Reptiles with erythroid regeneration or inflammation or with red blood cell bone marrow disorders may have increased anisocytosis and poikilocytosis, increased numbers of polychromatophils or more immature red blood cell precursors, increased irregularity of the nuclear membranes, basophilic stippling, binucleation, or mitoses (Figs. 12.3–12.5). Hypochromasia may be seen with iron deficiency. Intracytoplasmic inclusions may be caused by protozoal (hemogregarines; Fig. 12.6) or viral organisms (iridovirus). Hemogregarines are generally nonpathogenic and do not typically distort the host red blood cell. With few exceptions, other red blood cell proto-

Figure 12.4 Red blood cell mitosis. A binucleated red blood cell precursor with deep blue cytoplasm undergoing mitosis is in the center of the image. Another red blood cell precursor with irregular nuclear margins is in the right of the field. The small dots throughout the image are artifacts (dust particles). Green iguana (*Iguana iguana*) blood smear; quick stain; 100× objective.

zoa are considered incidental findings. Iridoviruses are pathogenic in infected reptiles and may form crystalline cytoplasmic inclusions in red blood cells. Infectious organisms must be differentiated from artifacts such as vacuolation (Figs. 12.7 and 12.8).

Figure 12.5 Poikilocytosis. Red blood cells with irregular nuclear membranes (in particular, the bottom right of the field), two thrombocytes (right and top of the field), and a teardrop red blood cell lacking a nucleus (bottom right) are shown. The inset is a greater magnification of an immature red blood cell with a ring-shaped nucleus from the same blood smear. This slide was overstained. Inland Bearded Dragon (*Pogona vitticeps*); quick stain; 100× objective.

Figure 12.6 Hemogregarine parasites. Two mature red blood cells contain single, intracytoplasmic, elongate, banana-shaped, blue protozoal gametocytes. Spiny-tailed lizard (*Uromastyx* sp.) blood smear; 100× objective.

NORMAL WHITE BLOOD CELL MORPHOLOGY

Heterophil

The heterophil of most reptilians has a cytoplasm that contains numerous elongate, generally oval- to rod- to spindle-shaped, orange to red-brown granules that may partially obscure the nucleus (Plate 4 [p. 95];

Figure 12.7 Red blood cell cytoplasmic vacuolation. The clear, variably sized, well-demarcated, cytoplasmic vacuoles in the red blood cells are artifacts. Lizard (unspecified genus) blood smear; 100× objective.

Figure 12.8 Red blood cell refractile artifact. The refractile amorphous, variably sized structures in the red blood cells are artifacts. Spiny-tailed lizard (*Uromastyx* sp.) blood smear; 100× objective.

Figs. 12.1 and 12.9). The size of the heterophil varies with the species of reptile and can vary in size from approximately 10 to 23 μm in diameter. In crocodilians, chelonians, and snakes, the nucleus of the mature heterophil has a round to oval shape (Plate 4; Fig. 12.9). In contrast, the nuclei of heterophils from lizards such as the green iguana (*Iguana iguana*) and the inland bearded dragon (*Pogona vitticeps*) are lobulated (Plate 4; Fig. 12.1). The lobulation is not as prominent as that of mammalian neutrophils. Heterophil granules may look less distinct with quick-stained blood smears when compared with Wright's stained blood smears.

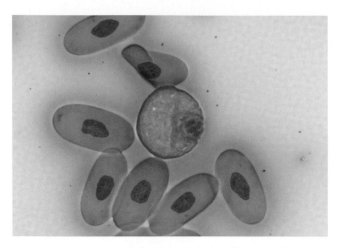

Figure 12.9 Heterophil. The round cell with abundant cytoplasm and a small, round, eccentrically located nucleus, filled with indistinct orange granules, is a mature heterophil. Boa snake (*Boa constrictor*) blood smear; 100× objective.

Figure 12.11 Lymphocytes. A small lymphocyte (top center of the field), a larger lymphocyte (top left of the field), and a heterophil are shown. Snake (unspecified genus) blood smear; 100× objective.

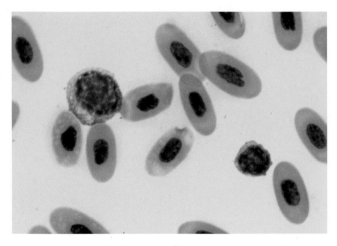

Figure 12.10 Lymphocytes. The round cells with single round nuclei and low amounts of blue cytoplasm are lymphocytes. A small lymphocyte (right of the field) and a larger lymphocyte (left of the field) are shown. Green iguana (*Iguana iguana*) blood smear; 100× objective.

Figure 12.12 Lymphocytes. Small (right image) and larger (left image) lymphocytes are shown in the center of each field. Green iguana (*Iguana iguana*) blood smear; quick stain; 100× objective.

Lymphocyte

In health, the lymphocyte is morphologically similar to that of mammals (Plate 4; Figures 12.10–12.14). Their size can range from approximately 5 to 15 μm in diameter. Within the same blood smear, there may be lymphocytes that are smaller and lymphocytes that are larger. Lymphocytes have single, eccentrically located round nuclei, low amounts of pale blue to blue cytoplasm, and high nuclear-to-cytoplasmic ratios. The chromatin is finely to coarsely clumped. Blood cells that may be confused at times with lymphocytes include thrombocytes (platelets) and immature red blood cells. Thrombocytes are typically oval, have very pale staining to nonstaining cytoplasm, and readily clump in blood smears (Figs. 12.13–12.15). Immature red blood cells that are round in shape may be confused with lymphocytes; however, lymphocytes have an eccentrically located nucleus versus the typical centrally located nucleus of the immature red blood cells, and lymphocytes generally have a higher nuclear-to-cytoplasmic ratio (i.e., lower amounts of cytoplasm relative to the size of the nucleus). The chromatin pattern of the immature red blood cells will be more similar to that of red blood cells (including polychromatophils) in the same smear. Significantly

Figure 12.13 Lymphocytes and thrombocytes. There are two lymphocytes and two thrombocytes (arrowheads). One lymphocyte is larger (left of the field) and has more cytoplasm than the smaller lymphocyte (bottom right of the field). Inland bearded dragon (*Pogona vitticeps*) blood smear; 100× objective.

Figure 12.15 Azurophil, lymphocyte, and thrombocyte. The round mononuclear cell with abundant pink-blue cytoplasm is an azurophilic monocyte (center of the field). The small round cell with a round nucleus and low amounts of blue cytoplasm is a small lymphocyte (bottom left of field). The small round mononuclear cell with a thin rim of blue cytoplasm is a thrombocyte (top of the field). Snake (unspecified genus) blood smear; 100× objective.

Figure 12.14 Monocyte, lymphocyte, and thrombocytes. The round mononuclear cell with abundant blue cytoplasm and round to oval nucleus is a monocyte (left of the field). The round cell with a round nucleus and scant amounts of cytoplasm is a small lymphocyte (top of the field). The clustered oval nucleated cells with scant amounts of blue cytoplasm are thrombocytes (bottom right of the field). Green iguana (*Iguana iguana*) blood smear; 100× objective.

Figure 12.16 Azurophils. The mononuclear round to oval cells with abundant blue to pink cytoplasm, a single round nucleus, and few cytoplasmic vacuoles are azurophilic monocytes (center of the field). Boa snake (*Boa constrictor*) blood smear; 100× objective.

increased numbers of polychromatophils should increase awareness that round, immature red blood cells may be present in the smear.

Monocyte

The monocyte of most reptilians is similar to that of mammals (Plate 4; Figs. 12.14–12.16). However, some monocytes of reptiles may have fine, dust-like pink granulation of the cytoplasm (Plate 4; Figs. 12.15 and 12.16). These cells are also referred to as azurophils or azurophilic monocytes. Monocytes are large mononuclear cells with abundant amounts of blue to blue-grey cytoplasm. Nuclei are oval to round and sometimes indented or U-shaped. Monocytes are generally larger, have less condensation of the chromatin than lymphocytes, and have a lower nuclear-to-cytoplasmic ratio. Monocytes may have a few clear cytoplasmic vacuoles.

Figure 12.17 Eosinophils and heterophils. The round mononuclear cell with numerous round cytoplasmic red granules and a round nucleus is an eosinophil (upper and lower images; center of the fields). Heterophils from the same tortoise are in the insets for comparison. The bottom image is from a blood smear stained with a quick stain; the upper image is from a blood smear of the same tortoise but stained with Wright's stain. Tortoise (unspecified genus) blood smear; 100× objective.

Figure 12.18 Eosinophil. The round mononuclear cell with pink to magenta cytoplasmic granules and an oval nucleus (center of the field) is an eosinophil. Boa snake (*Boa constrictor*) blood smear; 100× objective.

Figure 12.19 Eosinophils. The round mononuclear cells (right and left images) with bluish cytoplasmic granules are eosinophils. The blood smear shown in the left image was stained with a quick stain; the blood smear shown in the right image was stained with Wright's stain and was from the same animal. Green iguana (*Iguana iguana*); 100× objective.

Eosinophil

Eosinophils have colorless to pale blue cytoplasm that contains numerous round, bright red-orange to pink cytoplasmic granules; however, some reptile species such as the green iguana have eosinophil granules that are pale blue to gray (Plate 4; Fig. 12.17–12.19). The size of eosinophils varies according to the species of reptile and can range in size from approximately 9 to 20 μm in diameter. Lizards tend to have the smallest eosinophils, but this is not true for all lizards. Nuclei can be round to oval to mildly indented. Eosinophils with red-orange to pink granules may be differentiated from heterophils in the same blood smear by the shape (generally round in eosinophils) or the color

(more intense/bright color in eosinophils) of the granules.

Basophil

Basophils have numerous deep purple or magenta cytoplasmic granules that are generally round and small (Plate 4; Fig. 12.20). The granules may be so numerous as to obscure the nucleus. The size of reptilian basophils varies according to the species but can range in size from approximately 7 to 20 μm in diameter. A difference from the mammalian basophil is

Figure 12.20 Basophils. The two round to oval cells with dark purple cytoplasmic granules and small, clear cytoplasmic vacuoles are basophils (left and right of the field). Green iguana (*Iguana iguana*) blood smear; 100× objective.

that the nucleus of the basophil in reptiles is generally round to oval and not lobulated, as in mammals. The cytoplasm of reptilian basophils may sometimes look vacuolated or foamy; however, a few deep purple granules will still remain and may be easier to locate over the nucleus (Plate 4; Fig. 12.20).

VARIATIONS IN WHITE CELL MORPHOLOGY

Granulocytes

The range of granulocytic leukocyte morphologic abnormalities that can occur in reptiles in response to inflammatory and noninflammatory conditions is similar to that of mammals and includes heterophil left shifts, heterophil toxicity, giant heterophils, and rarely, mitoses in circulating leukocytes (Figs. 12.21–12.23). Similar to domestic species, left shift refers to the presence of immature heterophil precursors in the peripheral blood in response to an inflammatory insult that overwhelms the capacity of the bone marrow to respond (Figs. 12.21 and 12.22). Because heterophil precursors have decreased nuclear lobulation, left shifts are easier to identify in reptilian species that normally have lobulated heterophils in circulation, such as the green iguana and the inland bearded dragon. Band heterophils have a nonlobulated, U-shaped nucleus and cytoplasmic contents that may be similar to mature heterophils. Less mature precursors may have round to oval nuclei and darker blue cytoplasm and may have a mixture of rod-shaped gran-

Figure 12.21 Heterophil left shift and toxicity. Upper image: The five round cells with lobulated to oval nuclei, red cytoplasmic round to oval granules, and that are sometimes vacuolated are immature (left-shifted) and toxic heterophils. A large monocyte is in the center bottom of the field. Lower image: Three left-shifted heterophils (top and bottom center of the field), a monocyte, and a small lymphocyte are shown. The lower image was from a blood smear stained with a quick stain; the blood smear shown in the upper image was stained with Wright's stain and was from the same animal. Green iguana (*Iguana iguana*) blood smear; 100× objective.

ules and rounder granules. A few granules may be blue to purple. Heterophil toxicity typically manifests as darker blue cytoplasm, cytoplasmic foaminess, or vacuolation and may be accompanied by morphologic changes in the granules consisting of round shape or blue to purple colored granules side by side with the typical heterophil granules. Increased numbers of Döhle bodies, as occurs in mammals, does not appear to be a common finding of inflammation in reptiles. Giant heterophils may occur with inflammatory leukograms and manifests as larger-than-normal heterophils that have nuclear lobulation and typical heterophil granules (Fig. 12.22). Degranulation of

Figure 12.22 Heterophil left shift and toxicity. The three round cells with lobulated to round to oval nuclei, cytoplasmic red granules, and cytoplasmic vacuolation (bottom left and top right of the field) are immature and toxic heterophils. The lobulated heterophil in the right top of the field is larger ("giant") than a typical mature lobulated heterophil. Green iguana (*Iguana iguana*) blood smear; 100× objective.

Figure 12.24 Pyknosis. The cell in the center of the field with blue cytoplasm and few darkly staining spherical nuclear fragments is a pyknotic leukocyte. Eastern box turtle (*Terrapene carolina carolina*) blood smear courtesy of Dr. Michael M. Fry; 100× objective.

Figure 12.23 Leukocyte mitosis. The leukocyte at the bottom center of the field is a granulocyte undergoing mitosis. This may occur with inflammation and leukemia. There are five thrombocytes in the field also. Tokay gecko (*Gekko gecko*) blood smear; 100× objective.

Figure 12.25 Reactive lymphocyte. The round cell in the center of the field with a round nucleus, coarsely clumped chromatin, and dark blue cytoplasm is a reactive lymphocyte. Green iguana (*Iguana iguana*) blood smear; 100× objective.

granulocytes can also occur and results in clear distinct vacuoles in the cytoplasm of heterophils or other granulocytes (Fig. 12.22). Pyknotic leukocytes may occur in the peripheral blood with severe sepsis or viral infections (Fig. 12.24).

Lymphocytes and Monocytes

Reactive lymphocytes, plasma cells, increased pink cytoplasmic granulation of monocytes (azurophils), or increased monocyte vacuolation may occur in reptiles with inflammation or chronic antigenic stimulation (Figs. 12.25–12.28). Reactive lymphocytes have increased amounts of darker blue cytoplasm and may have a perinuclear clear zone (Figs. 12.25 and 12.26). Plasma cells may occur rarely and have abundant amounts of blue cytoplasm, perinuclear clear zones, Russell bodies, and dense eccentrically located nucleus (Fig. 12.27). Atypical or leukemic mononuclear cells (lymphocytic or monocytic) may occur with leukemia. Leukemic diseases are uncommon in reptiles.

Figure 12.26 Reactive plasmacytoid lymphocyte. The round cell in the top center of the field with a round, eccentrically located nucleus; coarsely clumped chromatin; dark blue cytoplasm; and perinuclear clear zone is a reactive plasmacytoid lymphocyte. Green iguana (*Iguana iguana*) blood smear; 100× objective.

Figure 12.27 Plasma cell. The round cell in the center of the field with a round nucleus, dark blue cytoplasm, eccentrically located nucleus, coarsely clumped chromatin, and a large pale blue cytoplasmic inclusion is a plasma cell with a Russell body (immunoglobulin accumulation). Green iguana (*Iguana iguana*) blood smear; 100× objective.

WHITE BLOOD CELL INCLUSIONS AND PARASITES

Inclusions in reptilian leukocytes are relatively infrequent findings. Inclusions are typically of infectious origin and include bacteria, viruses, or protozoa. Bacteria in leukocytes indicate severe sepsis/bacteremia and require immediate attention. Bacteria may occur within heterophils or monocytes. For example, *Chlamydophila* sp. (formerly known as *Chlamydia*) inclusions have been described in monocytes from a

Figure 12.28 Monocyte. The oval cell with an indented nucleus, blue cytoplasm, and numerous cytoplasmic clear vacuoles is a monocyte. Iguana (*Iguana iguana*) blood smear; 100× objective.

chameleon. Viral inclusions may be caused by poxviruses (eosinophilic lacy cytoplasmic inclusions in monocytes) and iridoviruses (eosinophilic cytoplasmic granular inclusions in heterophils and monocytes; Fig. 12.29). Protozoa include *Saurocytozoon* sp., *Schellackia* sp., and others. Lymphocytes, monocytes, or heterophils may be affected. Noninfectious causes of inclusions in leukocytes are uncommon.

THROMBOCYTE MORPHOLOGY IN HEALTH AND DISEASE

Thrombocytes of reptilians differ greatly from those of mammals. Reptilian thrombocytes are round to oval nucleated cells with colorless to pale staining cytoplasm and condensed round to oval nucleus (Figures 12.13–12.15 and 12.23). The size of thrombocytes varies from approximately 8 to 16 μm in their greatest dimension. The cytoplasm may also contain small vacuoles or pink granules, and they may be confused with small lymphocytes but can be differentiated from these cells on the basis of their generally oval shape, very pale staining to colorless cytoplasm, and tendency to frequently clump in blood smears.

Thrombocytes may undergo morphologic changes during disease. For example, nuclei may lose their round to oval shape and become variably shaped during inflammation. Inclusions may also occur within thrombocytes and are rarely caused by protozoa such as *Fallisia* sp and viruses such as poxvirus.

Figure 12.29 Iridoviral inclusions. Single, red, round, intracytoplasmic viral inclusions may occur in heterophils (upper image, arrowhead) and monocytes (lower image, arrowhead) of infected turtles. Eastern box turtle (*Terrapene carolina carolina*) blood smear courtesy of Dr. Michael M. Fry; 100× objective.

Figure 12.30 Microfilariae. The elongate, serpentine, sheathed organisms in the center of the field (upper and lower images) are microfilariae. The upper image was from a blood smear stained with a quick stain; the blood smear shown in the lower image was stained with Wright's stain and was from the same animal. Panther chameleon (*Furcifer paradalis*) blood smear; 100× objective.

EXTRACELLULAR BLOOD PARASITES AND OTHER CELLS

Microfilaria (Fig. 12.30), bacteria, and protozoa may occur in reptiles, particularly wild-caught pet reptiles from other localities, and local wildlife. Melanocytes or melanophages (macrophages with intracytoplasmic melanin) may occasionally occur in the blood of reptiles (Fig. 12.31).

Figure 12.31 Melanocyte or melanophage. The round cell with an oval nucleus and numerous brown cytoplasmic pigment granules is a melanocyte or melanophage. Green iguana (*Iguana iguana*) blood smear; 100× objective.

PLATE 4. Overview diagram of leukocytes in healthy reptiles. Heterophils typically have red to orange elongate cytoplasmic granules. Heterophils of lizards such as the green iguana (*Iguana iguana*) and the inland bearded dragon (*Pogona vitticeps*) have lobulated nuclei. In contrast, the nuclei of heterophils from snakes, turtles, tortoises, and crocodilians are round to oval. The granules may be so numerous that it may be difficult to see individual granules. Lymphocytes and monocytes are generally similar to those of domestic animals. Reptiles also have monocytes with pink, fine cytoplasmic granulation and are called azurophilic monocytes or azurophils (bottom cell of each pair of monocytes). Eosinophils generally have oval nuclei and round cytoplasmic granules. In some reptile species, such as some tortoises (T), the granules are pink to pale red, and in other reptile species, such as some snakes (S) and iguanas, the granules may have a blue to magenta hue. Basophils will have dark purple granules and may appear vacuolated.

Appendixes

Appendix 1: Semiquantitative Grading Scheme for Evaluation of Red Blood Cell Morphology*

Morphology and Species	Grading Scheme			
	1+	2+	3+	4+
Anisocytosis				
Dog	7–15	16–20	21–29	>30
Cat	5–8	9–15	16–20	>20
Cow	10–20	21–30	31–40	>40
Horse	1–3	4–6	7–10	>10
Polychromasia				
Dog	2–7	8–14	15–29	>30
Cat	1–2	3–8	9–15	>15
Cow	2–5	6–10	11–20	>20
Horse	. . . . rarely observed			
Hypochromasia				
All Species	1–10	11–50	51–200	>200
Poikilocytosis				
All Species	3–10	11–50	51–200	>200
Target Cells				
Dogs Only	3–5	6–15	16–30	>30
Spherocytes				
All Species	1–10	11–50	51–150	>150
Miscellaneous Morphology (Acanthocytes, Schistocytes, Dacryocytes, Heinz bodies, Howell-Jolly bodies, etc.)				
All Species	1–2	3–8	9–20	>20
Basophilic Stippling				
All Species	. . . . report as noted when observed			

Source: Adapted from Table 3 by Weiss, Douglass J. 1984. Uniform evaluation and semiquantitative reporting of hematologic data in veterinary laboratories. *Veterinary Clinical Pathology* 13(2):27–31. Permission granted by Wiley-Blackwell.

*Red blood cell morphology is assessed as the average number of abnormal cells in the monolayer of the smear using the 100× objective. When using this table, a monolayer is defined as a microscopic field in which approximately half of the red blood cells are touching each other.

APPENDIX 2: SEMIQUANTITATIVE GRADING SCHEME FOR EVALUATION OF NEUTROPHIL TOXICITY

Neutrophil toxicity*

1+ Mild basophilia

2+ Moderate basophilia and/or mild-foamy cytoplasm and Döhle bodies may be noted

3+ Marked basophilia and/or marked-foamy cytoplasm and Döhle bodies may be noted

4+ Criteria similar to 3+ with indistinct nuclear membranes

*In cats and horses, Döhle bodies may be present without other signs of toxicity; if so, the following classification would be used.

1+ <10% neutrophils contain Döhle bodies.

2+ 10 to 30% of neutrophils contain Döhle bodies.

3+ >30% of neutrophils contain Döhle bodies.

Glossary

Acanthocyte A red blood cell with multiple, variably sized, irregular membrane projections that are caused by alterations in the ratio of membrane cholesterol to phospholipids.

Antibodies A type of protein produced against antigens by the immune system.

Agglutination Clumping of red blood cells that is usually caused by cross-linking of red blood cell surface–associated antibodies.

Agranulocyte A white blood cell that does not contain secondary granules. The two types of agranulocytes are lymphocytes and monocytes.

Anemia A condition in which the hemoglobin, packed cell volume, and red blood cell count decrease below the normal reference range.

Anisocytosis A variation in the size of cells; in hematology, this is most often used to describe variation in the size of red blood cells.

Antigen A substance that can cause the immune system to produce antibodies.

Anticoagulant Substance that prevents the clotting of blood.

Azurophil See azurophilic monocyte.

Azurophilic granules Cytoplasmic granules that stain pink to reddish-purple with Wright's stain.

Azurophilic monocyte Monocyte of reptiles that contains many fine, dust-like cytoplasmic azurophilic granules. This cell is also referred to as an azurophil.

Band cell A type of white blood cell with a nuclear membrane that has parallel sides, although slight indentations may be present. Band cells can be of the neutrophilic, eosinophilic, or basophilic lineage.

Bar cell A red blood cell with a central, bar-shaped outfolding. This cell is also known as a knizocyte.

Basophil A white blood cell of the granulocytic lineage with a segmented nucleus, purple cytoplasm, and often purple cytoplasmic granules.

Basophilia The reaction of a cell to Wright's stain, resulting in a bluish-stained cytoplasm; also describes the color of the cytoplasm of toxic neutrophils or refers to an increase in the number of basophils in the circulation.

Basophilic A bluish color on Wright's-stained preparations; also refers to basophils.

Basophilic stippling The presence of very small, dark blue staining bodies within the red blood cell. The stippling is usually a result of RNA accumulation but may be associated with iron accumulation.

Binucleation Containing two nuclei.

Blister cell A red blood cell with a membrane vacuole.

Bone marrow The central portion of long, flat, and irregular bones that is the principal site of hematopoiesis.

Buffy coat A layer of white blood cells and platelets that collects immediately above the red blood cells in centrifuged whole blood; it has a whitish appearance.

Burr cell An oval to elongated red blood cell with multiple, fine projections.

Chelonian(s) Term used to refer to turtles, tortoises, or terrapins.

Chromatin A complex of DNA and nuclear proteins.

Codocyte A red blood cell with an extra round out-folding of membrane in the middle of the cell that gives the cell a target-like appearance. This cell is commonly known as a target cell.

Crenation An in vitro artifact that results in the formation of red blood cells with multiple, uniform, small, fine projections on the cell membrane.

Cytoplasm The portion of the cell that is exclusive of the nucleus.

Cytochemical A staining technique to identify cell types.

Dacryocyte A teardrop-shaped red blood cell that may be seen in animals with myelofibrosis.

Deoxyribonucleic acid (DNA) The nucleic acid that contains the basic genetic information found in the nuclei of cells.

Diff-Quik A commercially available preparation for manually staining slides with a modified Wright's stain.

Disseminated intravascular coagulation (DIC) A pathophysiological state that may develop as a result of damage of endothelial cells, activation of platelets, and activation of the coagulation system. This results in often severe, life-threatening, bleeding abnormalities.

Döhle body A small, round to irregular, blue structure in the cytoplasm of cells of the neutrophilic lineage. It is an abnormal aggregate of RNA in the cell and one sign of toxicity.

Dyserythropoiesis Myelodysplasia of cells of the erythrocytic lineage.

Dysgranulopoiesis Myelodysplasia of cells of the granulocytic lineage.

Dysthrombopoiesis Myelodysplasia of platelets.

Eccentrocyte A red blood cell with a crescent-shaped clear area that is eccentrically placed. This cell is formed as a result of oxidant-induced damage to the red blood cell membranes.

Echinocyte A red blood cell with multiple, small, delicate, regular-shaped spines distributed evenly around the membrane. The most common cause of echinocyte formation is an in vitro artifact known as crenation.

Eosinophil A white blood cell of the granulocytic lineage with reddish to reddish-orange granules in the cytoplasm.

Erythrocyte A mature red blood cell.

Erythropoiesis The production of red blood cells.

Ethylenediaminetetraacetate (EDTA) The antico-agulant most commonly used for the collection of blood for hematological examination.

Extracellular Located outside the cell.

Formalin A liquid used for preservation of tissues.

Ghost cell A remnant membrane of a red blood cell.

Granulocyte A white blood cell that contains secondary, also known as specific, cytoplasmic granules. The three different types of granulocytes are neutrophils, eosinophils, and basophils.

Granulopoiesis The production of granulocytes, which include cells of the neutrophilic, basophilic, and eosinophilic lineages.

Heterophil A granulocytic white blood cell that contains many orange to red, elongate to rod-shaped granules in the cytoplasm and is the counterpart of the neutrophil in reptiles and birds. This name is also used for the counterpart of the neutrophil in rabbits.

Heinz body A rounded, often refractile, projection from the surface of the red blood cell that is a result of oxidation and denaturation of hemoglobin.

Hematocrit The percentage of red blood cells relative to plasma.

Hematology The study of blood.

Hematopoiesis The production of blood cells.

Hemoglobin The protein in red blood cells that carries oxygen.

Hemosiderin The insoluble form of iron that appears as golden-brown to black, granular to globular material.

Heparin A type of anticoagulant.

Howell-Jolly body A small piece of remnant nuclear material in the red blood cell.

Hypochromasia The presence of red blood cells in the circulation that have increased central pallor and decreased staining intensity of the membrane as a result of a decreased hemoglobin content.

Hypochromic cell A red blood cell with increased central pallor and decreased staining intensity of the membrane.

Immunophenotyping Characteristics of cells determined by immunological reagents.

Karyorrhexis Disruption of the cell nucleus, resulting in multiple fragments.

Keratocyte A red blood cell with two fairly uniform hornlike projections.

Knizocyte A red blood cell with a central, bar-shaped outfolding. This cell is also known as a bar cell.

Kurloff body A large eosinophilic inclusion found in guinea pig lymphocytes.

Left shift An increase in the number of band neutrophils and other immature cells of the granulocytic lineage in the peripheral blood.

Leptocyte A red blood cell, which, typically, is larger, with excessive, thin membranes and folds easily. Target cells and bar cells are types of leptocytes.

Leukemia A neoplastic proliferation of cells of bone marrow origin that are usually released into the blood.

Leukemic Pertaining to leukemia

Leukemoid Pertaining to the presence of very high numbers of neutrophilic granulocytes in the circulation, often with many immature forms; caused by the degree of elevation of the white blood cell count, this may be confused with a true leukemia.

Leukocyte A white blood cell.

Lobulation A structure divided into lobes, which are rounded projections.

Lymphocyte A white blood cell of the agranulocytic lineage that is characterized by a round nucleus and light blue cytoplasm. There are two main types: B lymphocytes, which develop into plasma cells and produce antibodies, and T lymphocytes, which are important in the cellular immune response.

Lymphoproliferative disorder A clonal neoplastic proliferation of cells of the lymphocytic lineage.

Macrocyte A red blood cell that is larger than normal.

Macrophage A large phagocytic cell found in tissues such as the bone marrow; this cell develops from a blood monocyte.

Mast cell A granulated round cell found in low numbers in the bone marrow.

Medullary Pertaining to bone marrow.

Megakaryocyte A very large cell that produces platelets and is found in the bone marrow.

Metamyelocyte The stage of development of granulocytes between the myelocyte and the band cell.

Metarubricyte The stage of development of red blood cells between the rubricyte and the polychromatophil.

Mitotic cell A cell that is undergoing division; the chromosomes are visible.

Monocyte A white blood cell of the agranulocytic lineage that is characterized by a variably shaped nucleus and blue-gray cytoplasm, which is frequently vacuolated.

Myeloblast The cell that is the earliest microscopically identifiable stage of development of granulocytes found in the bone marrow.

Myelocyte The stage of development of granulocytes between the promyelocyte and the metamyelocyte.

Myelodysplasia Alterations in the normal development and maturation of cells of the myeloid lineage.

Myelofibrosis A condition in which the bone marrow has varying degrees of increased fibrous connective tissue that displaces the normal blood cell precursors.

Myeloid   Pertaining to the bone marrow. More specifically, this term is used to collectively describe the cells of the granulocytic, erythrocytic, megakaryocytic, and monocytic lineages.

Myeloproliferative disorder   A clonal neoplastic proliferation of cells of the myeloid lineage.

Neutrophil   A white blood cell of the granulocytic lineage with a segmented nucleus and pink to light blue cytoplasm.

New methylene blue stain   A stain used to identify reticulocytes and to more readily see Heinz bodies.

Nonregenerative anemia   An anemia in which there is not adequate production of red blood cells in the bone marrow.

Nucleolus   A small round structure in the nuclei of cells that contains RNA and protein; it usually stains bluish with Wright's stain. Nucleoli (pl.).

Nucleus   The central spherical structure within a cell that contains DNA, nucleoli, and nuclear proteins. Nuclei (pl.).

Osteoblast   A cell found in low numbers in the bone marrow. It is important in bone formation.

Osteoclast   A very large multinucleated cell in the bone marrow that is important in bone remodeling.

Ovalocyte   An oval-shaped red blood cell.

Packed cell volume (PCV)   The percentage of red blood cells relative to plasma, determined by centrifugation.

Pappenheimer bodies   Iron inclusions in red blood cells that appear as pale blue granules with Wright's stain.

Polymerase chain reaction (PCR)   Technique involving amplification of specific nucleic acid sequences (DNA or RNA).

Plasma   The fluid noncellular portion of anticoagulated whole blood.

Plasma cell   An oval cell with eccentric nuclei; it may be found in the bone marrow and produces antibodies.

Platelet   A small, anucleated cytoplasmic fragment from megakaryocytes that is present in the peripheral blood and is important in hemostasis. This cell is also known as a thrombocyte.

Poikilocytosis   The presence of abnormally shaped red blood cells in the circulation.

Polychromasia   The presence of polychromatophils in the blood.

Polychromatophil   An immature red blood cell that is typically larger than the mature red blood cell and stains bluish to bluish-red with Wright's stain.

Promyelocyte   The stage of development of granulocytes between the myeloblast and the myelocyte.

Prorubricyte   The stage of development of red blood cells between the rubriblast and the rubricyte.

Punched-out cell   A red blood cell with accentuated central pallor. This cell is also known as a torocyte.

Pyknotic cell   A cell with a small nucleus and very condensed chromatin.

Reactive lymphocyte   A lymphocyte with a dark blue cytoplasm and, sometimes, a perinuclear clear zone. Also, the cell may be larger than a typical small lymphocyte.

Red blood cell (RBC)   An anucleated cell that stains reddish to reddish-orange with Wright's stain. The main function of the red blood cell is to carry oxygen.

Regenerative anemia   An anemia in which there is an increase in production of red blood cells in the bone marrow, with subsequent release into the peripheral blood.

Reticular   Resembling a net.

Reticulocyte   An immature erythrocyte that contains clumps of ribosomal RNA and mitochondria, which stain with new methylene blue. These cells correspond to polychromatophils seen in Wright's-stained preparations.

Ribonucleic acid (RNA) The nucleic acid that is important in protein synthesis.

Rough endoplasmic reticulum A cytoplasmic organelle that is important in protein synthesis.

Rouleaux Organized linear arrays and sometimes branching chains of red blood cells.

Rubriblast The cell that is the earliest microscopically identifiable stage of development of red blood cells found in the bone marrow.

Rubricyte A stage of development of red blood cells between the prorubricyte and the metarubricyte.

Schistocyte An irregularly shaped fragment of a red blood cell.

Sideroblast A nucleated red blood cell that contains Pappenheimer bodies.

Siderocyte An anucleated red blood cell that contains Pappenheimer bodies.

Sodium citrate A type of anticoagulant.

Smudge cell A cell with no intact cell membrane but only free nuclear chromatin material. This cell is sometimes called a basket cell because of the delicate, woven, basket-like strands of dispersed nuclear chromatin.

Spherocyte A smaller-appearing red blood cell that lacks central pallor and is usually a result of immune-mediated damage to the cell.

Stomatocyte A red blood cell with central pallor that is oval to elongated and takes on the appearance of a mouth.

Target cell A red blood cell with an extra round outfolding of membrane in the middle of the cell that gives the cell a target-like appearance. This cell is also known as a codocyte.

Thrombocyte In mammals it refers to a small, anucleated cytoplasmic fragment from a megakaryocyte that is present in the peripheral blood and important in hemostasis. In reptiles and birds, thrombocytes are nucleated and have the same general function as thrombocytes in mammals. Thrombocytes are also known as platelets.

Torocyte A red blood cell with accentuated central pallor. This cell is commonly known as a punched-out cell.

Toxicity A group of morphological changes during inflammation that may be present in cells of the neutrophilic lineage. The three main features of toxicity are increased basophilia, foaminess, and the presence of Döhle bodies in the cytoplasm.

White blood cell (WBC) A nucleated cell in the blood that does not contain hemoglobin. This cell is also known as a leukocyte. The two major types of white blood cells are granulocytes and agranulocytes.

SELECTED REFERENCES

Alleman, A.R., and J.W. Harvey. 1993. The morphologic effects of vincristine sulfate on canine bone marrow cells. *Veterinary Clinical Pathology* 22(2): 36–41.

Bolliger, A.P. 2004. Cytological evaluation of bone marrow in rats: indications, methods, and normal morphology. *Veterinary Clinical Pathology* 33(2): 58–67.

Campbell, T.W., and C.K. Ellis. 2007. *Avian and exotic animal hematology & cytology*, 3rd ed. Ames, IA: Blackwell Publishing.

Cowell R.L., R.D. Tyler, J.H. Meinkoth, and D.B. DeNicola. 2008. *Diagnostic cytology and hematology of the dog and cat*. 3rd ed. St. Louis, MO: Mosby.

Duncan, J.R., K.W. Prasse, and E.A. Mahaffey. 1994. *Veterinary laboratory medicine: clinical pathology*, 3rd ed. Ames: Iowa State University Press.

Feldman B.F., J.G. Zinkl, and N.C. Jain, 2000. *Schalm's veterinary hematology*, 5th ed. Baltimore: Lippincott, Williams & Wilkins.

Fox, J.C., S.A. Ewing, R.G. Buckner, D. Whitenack, and J.H. Manley. 1986. *Trypanosoma cruzi* infection in a dog from Oklahoma. *Journal of the American Veterinary Medical Association* 189(12): 1583–4.

Fyfe, J.C., P.F. Jezyk, U. Giger, and D.F. Patterson. 1989. Inherited selective malabsorption of vitamin B12 in giant schnauzers. *Journal of the American Animal Hospital Association* 25: 533–9.

Glenn, B.L., and E.L. Stair. 1984. Cytauxzoonosis in domestic cats: Report of two cases in Oklahoma, with a review and discussion of the disease. *Journal of the American Veterinary Medical Association* 184(7): 822–5.

Hall R.L., and N.E. Everds. 2003. Factors affecting the interpretation of canine and non-human primate clinical pathology. *Toxicological Pathology* 31(Suppl): 6–10.

Harvey, J.W. 2001. *Atlas of veterinary hematology: blood and bone marrow of domestic animals*. Philadelphia: Saunders.

Jain, N.C. 1986. *Schalms veterinary hematology*, 4th ed. Philadelphia: Lea and Febiger.

Jain, N.C. 1993. *Essentials of veterinary hematology*. Philadelphia: Lea and Febiger.

Latimer, K.S. 1995. Leukocytes in health and disease. In *Textbook of veterinary internal medicine: diseases of the dog and cat*, 4th ed., ed. Stephen J. Ettinger and Edward C. Feldman, 1892–1929. Philadelphia: W.B. Saunders.

Latimer, K.S., E.A. Mahaffey, and K.W. Prasse. 2003. *Duncan and Prasse's veterinary laboratory medicine: clinical pathology*, 4th ed. Ames, IA: Blackwell Publishing.

Messick, J.B. 2004. Hemotrophic mycoplasmas (hemoplasmas): a review and new insights into pathogenic potential. *Veterinary Clinical Pathology* 33(1): 2–13.

Myers, S., K. Wiks, and U. Giger. 1995. Macrocytic anemia caused by naturally-occurring folate-deficiency in the cat. *Veterinary Pathology* 32(5): 547.

Reagan, W.J., and A.H. Rebar. 1995. Platelet disorders. In *Textbook of veterinary internal medicine: diseases of the dog and cat*, 4th ed., ed. Stephen J. Ettinger and Edward C. Feldman, 1964–1976. Philadelphia: W.B. Saunders.

Reagan, W.J., F. Garry, M.A. Thrall, S. Colgan, J. Hutchison, and M.G. Weiser. 1990. The clinicopathologic, light, and scanning electron microscopic features of eperythrozoonosis in four naturally infected llamas. *Veterinary Pathology* 27: 426–31.

Rebar, A.H., P.S. MacWilliams, B.F. Feldman, F.L. Metzger, R.V.H. Pollock, and J. Roche. 2001. *Guide to hematology in dogs and cats*. Jackson, WY: Teton New Media.

Rich, Lon J. 1976. *The morphology of canine and feline blood cells*. St. Louis, MO: Ralston Purina Company.

Strik, N.I., et al. 2007. Circulating inflammatory cells. In *Infectious diseases and pathology of reptiles, color atlas and text*, pp. 167–218. Boca Raton, FL: CRC Press.

Taboada, J., and S.R. Merchant. 1995. Protozoal and miscellaneous infections. In *Textbook of veterinary internal medicine: diseases of the dog and cat*, 4th ed., ed. Stephen J. Ettinger and Edward C. Feldman, 384–97. Philadelphia: W.B. Saunders.

Thrall, M.A., D.C. Baker, T.W. Campbell, D.B. DeNicola, M.J. Fettman, D.E. Lassen, A. Rebar, and G. Weiser. 2006. *Veterinary hematology and clinical chemistry; text and clinical case presentations*. Ames, IA: Blackwell Publishing.

Van Houten, D., M.G. Weiser, L. Johnson, and F. Garry. 1992. Reference hematologic values and morphologic features of blood cells in healthy adult llamas. *American Journal of Veterinary Research* 53(10): 1773–79.

Weiser, M.G. 1995. Erythrocyte responses and disorders. In *Textbook of veterinary internal medicine: diseases of the dog and cat*, 4th ed., ed. Stephen J. Ettinger and Edward C. Feldman, 1864–91. Philadelphia: W.B. Saunders.

Weiss, D.J. 1984. Uniform evaluation and semiquantitative reporting of hematologic data in veterinary laboratories. *Veterinary Clinical Pathology* 13(2): 27–31.

Willard, M.D., H. Tvedten, and G.H. Turnwald. 1989. *Small animal clinical diagnosis by laboratory methods*. Philadelphia: W.B. Saunders.

INDEX

Bold numbers indicate figures